DEVELOPMENTS IN THE
SUPERVISION
of MIDWIVES

DEVELOPMENTS IN THE
SUPERVISION
of MIDWIVES

Editor:
Mavis Kirkham

Authors:
Mavis Kirkham PhD, RM, RGN, BA, MA, CERT ED
Gill Halksworth RGN, RM, BA (HONS), MN, MSC
Barbara Bale RGN, RM, ADM, PGCEA, MSC
Chris James BSC, PhD
Jean Duerden MBA, RN, RSCN, RM
Helen Stapleton MSC, SRN, SCM, MNIMH
Olive Jones RGN, RM, RSCN, RHV, DIP IN HEALTH ETHICS
Frances Derbyshire RGN, RM, PGCERT, ADM
Glynnis Mayes MSC, BSC, RGN, RM, RHV
Cathy Rogers MA, RM, RMN, RN, ADM, PGCEA
Chris Hallworth RM, RN, MTD

Books *for* **Midwives Press**

Published by Books for Midwives Press
Oxford Road, Manchester, England.

ISBN 1 898507 78 3

A catalogue record for this book is
available from the British Library.

Printed in Great Britain by Redwood Books Ltd.

Introduction

There has been much recent work on the supervision of midwives and there have been considerable changes in the context of supervision. This book is concerned with these developments and follows on from *Supervision of Midwives* (Kirkham, 1996).

The first large studies of supervision of midwives in England and in Wales were carried out in 1996-7 and these are outlined in the first section of this book (Chapters 1-4). Chapter 1 outlines the research of Gill Halksworth, Barbara Bale and Chris James to evaluate the supervision of midwives in Wales. Chapters 2-4 outline the research on supervision in England carried out by Helen Stapleton, Jean Duerden and myself. Jean Duerden's audit of supervision is included here (Chapter 2) as it was carried out as part of that research project. The central section of the book is concerned with changes in the practice of supervision. It says a lot about the desire to improve supervision that this section opens (Chapter 5) with details of the early implementation of the research reported in the earlier chapters. One clear and important change in England and Wales is towards midwives choosing their supervisor. It is unusual, and very cheering, for research to be heeded and efforts made to implement its findings so rapidly.

Jean Duerden documents the new local supervising authority (LSA) arrangements in Chapter 6. This chapter covers all of the UK and includes an examination of the LSA role in clinical governance. Yet such is the speed of change, that the chapter ends by questioning what will happen to these arrangements with the impending changes in the statutory bodies.

Chapters 7 and 8 concern examples of innovation in supervision. Olive Jones writes on developing a framework for supervision in a midwife managed birth centre in Edgware (Chapter 7). Frances Derbyshire writes on clinical supervision within midwifery in the neonatal unit in Exeter (Chapter 8). Each of these, very different, chapters demonstrates the implementation of strategies for personal and professional development which involve midwives experiencing power sharing, guided by supervisors who consciously model such empowerment. In each case the aim is the parallel empowerment of clients, enhancing their care through enhancing the care experienced by their carers.

Chapter 9 consists of three anonymised case studies of supervision. These are included as food for thought and to reflect both developments and dilemmas in supervision. Case Study 1, concerned with a midwife's care of her childbearing daughter, includes the new West Midlands LSA's *Regional Guidance for Supervisors of Midwives When Receiving Requests from Midwives to Deliver Relatives or Friends*. This is a timely document acknowledging the support needed when personal and professional relationships come together.

The final section of the book is concerned with education for supervisors. In Chapter 10, Glynnis Mayes describes the development of the new ENB distance learning package. The original distance learning package was widely acknowledged as being a vast improvement in the preparation of supervisors (Stapleton et al, 1998 and Chapter 10). Chapter 10 is concerned with the development of the 1997 package and its evaluation. In Chapter 11 Cathy Rogers and Chris Hallworth describe the development of the preparation of supervisors at Masters level at the University of Hertfordshire. This was the first such course at Masters level. This academic development acknowledges the depth of both the analytical thinking and interpersonal skills required of supervisors.

The context of supervision continues to change. Nationwide changes in the organisation of the NHS led to the changes in the LSAs described by Jean Duerden in Chapter 5. Changes in professional regulation and the statutory bodies, not published as this book goes to press, will lead to further changes in the organisation and future of supervision.

Within NHS maternity units, many changes have influenced supervision and created new dilemmas. Midwifery management posts have been cut and many new supervisors are not managers. These changes, together with improvements in the education of supervisors, should lessen past confusions between management and supervisory roles. Midwives want supervisors who are accessible and who understand their clinical situation, yet they also want supervisors who can exercise 'clout' on behalf of midwives (Chapters 3 and 4). It may well be that making supervisors more accessible creates a need to rethink how leadership 'clout' is best achieved.

Midwives who are not NHS employees have experienced particular problems around supervision from supervisors who are also managers within the NHS (Demilew 1996 and Stapleton et al 1998). In 1998 the first supervisors of midwives outside the NHS were appointed. We await with interest the impact these supervisors will make.

Changes in the ethos of the NHS also influence supervision. Recent emphasis upon audit, quality standards and clinical guidelines has created a climate where supervision of midwives can be demonstrated as a mechanism very relevant to contemporary practice. Chapter 7 provides an example of a supervisor facilitating the development of guidelines in a way which was flexible and attentive to individuals and which resulted in the midwives feeling ownership of appropriate guidelines. A flexibility and sensitivity in practice was developed that 'avoids imposing routines which may lead to depersonalised care'. Such a situation clearly followed a parallel process in the care midwives received in supervision.

Such flexibility is, however, not always achieved. Audit, risk management and other monitoring techniques can be used rigidly and inflexibly. Glynnis Mayes (Chapter 11) warns against risk management being implemented in 'a controlling and restrictive fashion'. At its best, the supervision of midwives demonstrates how monitoring of quality can be achieved in a manner which practitioners find enhances their practice and their confidence.

Changing the culture of midwifery in the NHS remains a real challenge (Chapter 3). It may be that the emphasis upon primary care, with the development of midwifery within primary care groups may provide opportunities for cultural change. Care in supportive community teams could provide opportunities for collaborative practice development and professional change which are difficult to achieve within institutions. Similarly, in a small setting offering midwife led care, it is possible for supervisors to facilitate cultural change towards empowerment for midwives and clients (Chapter 7). This is not to say that such change cannot be achieved within large institutions and this book contains many different examples of work towards that end.

Perhaps the biggest imminent change in the context of supervision is clinical governance. Clinical governance is defined as:

a framework through which NHS organisations are accountable for continuously improving the quality of their services and safeguarding high standards of care by creating an environment in which excellence in clinical care will flourish. (NHSE 1999)

This must be entirely congruent with the long-established aims of the supervision of midwives. In this sense midwifery has the advantage of an existing and established structure to achieve these aims. This is described in Chapter 6. The dilemmas in the practice of supervision are also foreseen for clinical governance:

Above all, clinical governance is about changing organisational culture in a systematic and demonstrable way, moving away from a culture of 'blame' to one of learning so that quality infuses all aspects of the organisation's work. (NHSE 1999)

There is no doubt that the culture of blame can greatly limit the effectiveness of supervision in midwifery. Yet supervisors can create a 'thinking environment' and act as a 'sounding board' for ongoing learning (Chapter 7). The importance of such a sounding board was raised by midwives in Wales (Chapter 1). Chapter 7 describes a process where guided reflection facilitated by a supervisor resulted in midwives feeling both supported and stretched with resulting increases in professional confidence and effective communication. Similar achievements in supervision were recorded in one of the sites researched in England (Chapters 3 and 4). In Case Study 2 (Chapter 9) the supervisor acknowledges the importance of 'changing the culture':

So the process by which we do things... like critical incident investigation is really, really important because that's one way we can bring home to everyone that changing the culture can make a difference. It's about being honest and saying that nobody can guarantee a particular outcome... (Case Study 2, Chapter 9)

It is noteworthy that this was said in the context of a critical incident where the culture of blame is often evident. It was also said in a large maternity unit, though cultural change is probably easier to achieve in smaller settings where fewer individuals and professions are involved.

Educational change is also evident within supervision, which may well result from advances in the education of supervisors (Chapters 10 and

11). The educational skills now needed by supervisors are considerable. Chapter 7 describes a supervisor facilitating reflection on practice with very positive results. A supervisor described in the English research (Chapter 3) as having exemplary skill in challenging and empowering midwives was a lecturer practitioner and certainly demonstrated educational skill in her supervisory role. Progress is also being made in the use of learning contracts following critical incidents (Chapter 4). They are used in Case Studies 2 and 3 (Chapter 9). Appropriate design and use of learning contracts requires considerable educational skill, as the supervisor in Case Study 2 (Chapter 9) stated:

> ... *supervising someone through the process of a learning contract is hard work because it means pressing that person to engage at a different level and to embed the learning a bit more at a practice level.*

Whilst this may not always be successful, it carries considerable potential, not least for uniting theory and practice.

The ENB publication *Supervision in Action: a practical guide for midwives* (ENB, 1999) is a direct result of our research in England which should prove useful in the education of midwives regarding supervision.

It is clear from the research in England and Wales that midwives think that their supervision influences their practice. This influence is not always positive. There are, however, many positive examples in this book of innovations in supervision and of innovations in linked fields such as the introduction of clinical supervision for midwives in the neonatal unit in Exeter (Chapter 8). Where supervisors work with flexibility, skill, and a desire to share power with midwives, their influence is profound and midwives are equipped to relate similarly with their clients. This book aims to illustrate some of these processes and to be useful to supervisors seeking to create strategies for good supervision. We also aim to give a picture of supervision as it responds to a rapidly changing world.

This book is the result of the efforts of many people. The authors of chapters are to be thanked for their contributions. I would especially like to thank those who cannot be named but without whom this book would have been not be possible: the anonymous contributors to the case studies in Chapter 9 and all those who contributed to the research in

England and Wales. Thanks are also due to those who provided information on the new LSA arrangements in Chapter 6. Last, but never least, I thank Jane Durell whose quiet and cheerful efficiency facilitates our work in the Women's Informed Childbearing and Health Research Group, University of Sheffield.

Mavis Kirkham

References

Demilew, J. (1996). 'Independent Midwives' View of Supervision'. In: Kirkham M (ed.) *Supervision of Midwives*. Hale: Books for Midwives Press.

ENB (1999). *Supervision in Action: A practical guide for midwives*. London: ENB.

Kirkham, M. (ed.) (1996). *Supervision of Midwives*. Hale: Books for Midwives Press.

NHS Executive (1999). *Clinical Governance: Quality in the new NHS*. London: HMSO.

Stapleton, H., Duerden, J. and Kirkham, M. (1998). *Evaluation of the Impact of the Supervision of Midwives on Professional Practice and the Quality of Midwifery Care*. London: ENB.

Gill Halksworth • Barbara Bale • Chris James

Evaluation of Supervision of Midwives

Wales

RESEARCH AND AUDIT

This chapter relates to the supervision of midwives in Wales during the period of May 1996 to April 1997. Whilst gathering the data it became apparent that the supervision of midwives in Wales was indeed changing and we were in actual fact 'standing on shifting sand' as the project was being conducted. Not only was the role of the supervisor at the clinical level changing but the changes brought about by the Health Authorities Act meant that the role of the lead supervisor was also being reviewed and adapting to the changing climate.

The following gives an overview of the methods used for the research, the data gleaned and some implications suggested by the results. It is hoped that the information gathered and the results presented will be of benefit for future practice and research and possibly for the training of supervisors of midwives. The outcomes could contribute not only to the improvement of professional midwifery practice; because of the nature of midwifery supervision and its legislative context, they could also inform practice in other health care professions, particularly in the light of the introduction of clinical supervision and clinical governance.

Background

The supervision of midwifery has a long history dating back to the first attempts to license midwives in the fifteenth century; Kirkham (1995) has given a succinct overview of the development of the role which therefore will not be repeated here. Suffice it to say that the Midwifery Act of 1902 established the current statutory framework for supervision; subsequent changes in legislation, policy and particularly practice have additionally influenced its nature. The history of midwifery has always encompassed conflict about the purpose and scope of supervision. The 'policing' dimension has invariably been a dominant influence and this aspect of supervision continues to be a very problematic area causing tension for some practising midwives and supervisors (for example Walton, 1995; Leap and Hunter, 1993; Kargar, 1993; Flint, 1985). However, there is a movement towards a more proactive, supportive, yet challenging role for supervisors (Mayes, 1995). This approach is seen to be more responsive to midwives' needs, and incorporates the notion of empowerment, the facilitation of professional development and potential improvement in practice.

In recent years, maternity services throughout the UK have been the focus of much attention. Recommendations have been made in each of the four countries regarding the practice of good maternity care, particularly in terms of effectiveness and efficiency. The *Protocol for Investment in Health Gain: Maternal and Early Child Health* (WHPF, 1991), hereafter referred to as the Protocol, is the guiding document in Wales. It sets out a number of health gain and service targets, some of which could be directly affected by supervision. The question naturally arises as to whether there are different ways of undertaking supervision which have more effect on practice and on meeting the service targets.

The project

Research was undertaken as a ground-clearing exercise to provide descriptive material as to the practice of supervisors in Wales. The work within the project was broadly divided into two phases: the survey phase and the case study phase.

The survey phase had two parts. The first related to all supervisors in Wales and the second specifically focused on the lead supervisors. 'Lead' supervisors in Wales are those who advise the local supervising authority, which is now the health authority, on midwifery issues and 'link' supervisors have evolved at trust level for ease of communication between the lead supervisor and the supervisors within each trust. In the first part of the survey phase a postal questionnaire was sent to all the practising supervisors of midwives in Wales (n=59) which attracted a 93 per cent response rate. The purpose of this questionnaire was to explore both the structure of supervision in place and the role and functions of the supervisors themselves.

The purpose of the survey of lead supervisors was to explore their specific role and responsibilities. The 1995 Health Authorities Act resulted in a restructuring of the local supervising authorities (LSAs) and had implications for the lead supervisors. Therefore, we undertook a telephone survey prior to the Act and a focus group nine months after the Act had been implemented.

The second phase involved gathering data in a number of case study areas (n=5). This related to a more in-depth study of supervision in specific areas, with both supervisors and midwives participating in semi-structured interviews (a total of 38 interviews were undertaken in the case study areas). The purpose of this phase of the research was to explore the structure and function of supervision from the perspectives of both supervisors and midwives. In addition, the research aimed to explore the contemporary practice of supervision in order to establish its impact on practice, particularly in relation to the achievement of targets within the Protocol (WHPF, 1991).

For the purposes of this chapter the data from these two phases regarding the views of supervisors and midwives are presented together with the latter section reporting on the survey of the lead supervisor. For a more detailed account of the results the full project report is available.

The results

The role and function of supervision

In terms of the structure of supervision the range and experience of the supervisors was sought. The mean length of time that the respondents had been in post as a supervisor was three years and seven months, with a range of less than one year to sixteen years. However, more than half (58 per cent) had been supervisors for less than two years.

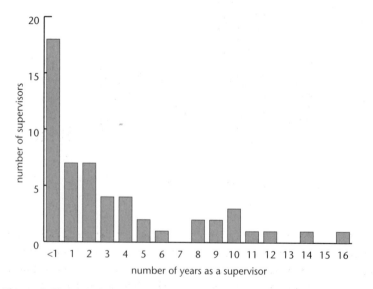

Figure 1: The duration of the experience of the respondents as supervisors

Selection for the post had in the past generally been by nomination or being asked to take on this role. The alternative method of selection was following an interview and eight supervisors had been selected by this method. There appeared to be a gradual move away from nomination and toward a more open selection. This has resulted recently in more clinicians, rather than purely managers, being appointed to supervisory posts. Many of the midwives interviewed were unsure of how supervisors came into post, while others were more certain and reiterated the information given by the supervisors. Some were critical and possibly cynical about the selection process. For example, one respondent considered that 'it depends on who you are friendly with'. In all areas, consideration was being given to alternative methods of appointing supervisors, with election of supervisors being suggested by some as a possibility for the future.

The employed position of supervisors

The grades at which supervisors are employed are illustrated in Figure 2. This graph shows the move toward employing clinically based midwives (in the main G, H, I grades) as well as managers (SMP).

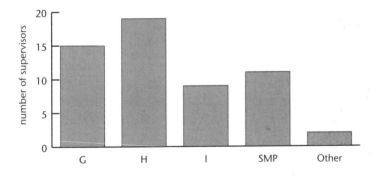

Figure 2: The clinical grades of the supervisors

To discern more accurately the positions held by the supervisors, the responses for the questions relating to the employed position and grading were cross-referenced. This revealed that 76 per cent of respondents held a management role, or by the nature of their job undertook management duties, with 33 per cent having dual roles i.e. clinical and managerial responsibilities.

The dual responsibility – as a supervisor and in their employed position – caused difficulties for some (Figure 3). Only ten people said that they had no difficulty at all in managing their dual responsibilities, with a minority identifying a substantial difficulty. Clearly, there is a problem to be faced here.

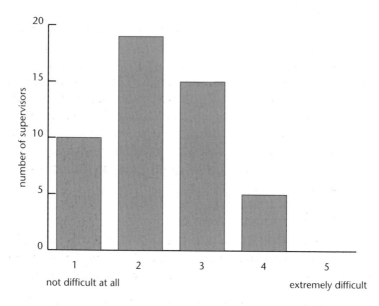

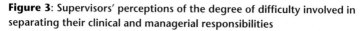

Figure 3: Supervisors' perceptions of the degree of difficulty involved in separating their clinical and managerial responsibilities

The mean ratio of supervisor to midwives at the time of the study was 1:31. However, it ranged from 1:12 to 1:98 (albeit during absence of supervisors due to sickness). Nine per cent of respondents had a ratio above the recommended level of 1:40 (UKCC, 1993 and 1998). Practice in the allocation of midwives to supervisors varied, although in only nine per cent of cases did the midwives themselves have a choice. More commonly, allocation was according to the area of work or at random, with a minority of supervisors choosing individual midwives. Comments were made by some that the method of allocation was going to change: '[there is] no choice at present but midwives will be given the choice in the future'.

The roles adopted by the supervisors

The supervisors interpreted their role in a variety of ways. Although there was no clearly articulated model evident, many of the activities they stated were associated with the 'normative role' – the monitoring and quality aspects as described in the model defined by Proctor (1986) (please see the glossary at the end of this chapter for a description of the roles as described by Proctor). These activities remained the key statutory functions and a significant priority for the supervisors.

However, interestingly, it became apparent that supervisors spent a greater proportion of their time on the formative and restorative, rather than on the normative functions, in day-to-day supervisory practice. Activities undertaken by the supervisors suggested that they spent most of their time either supporting midwives in their practice, or in carrying out their development/formative work. Although protection of the public remained their priority function, how this was enacted obviously varied on an individual basis. Certainly when asked about dealing with situations when the safety of mother and baby had been jeopardised it was clear that cases had been detected although these were in the minority.

The practice of supervision

The supervisory role was carried out in a variety of ways. The monitoring role was a predominant method of assessing the quality of midwives' work and was seen as being crucial for some supervisors:

> I look at their work, I work with them, I follow up the women's notes to see what is being documented and what the midwives are doing and we have an informal interview every year.

Other supervisors wanted to move away from the 'monitoring, punitive' side of supervision:

> There will always be incidents where maybe the midwife didn't act quite as she should have, but I would rather not think of it as being punitive in that way but supporting – identifying a problem and working with her and supporting her to ensure she has the confidence to continue.

Other midwives acknowledged that supervisors have a principal role in upholding clinical standards:

> *She's your colleague and she's possibly your mentor... she ensures that we give a good standard of care and maintain a high standard.*

The manner in which the supervisors ensured the quality of care delivered varied in each area and was often dependent on the nature of their employed position. For example, a supervisor with combined responsibilities as a manager observed practice as these midwives describe:

> *They just come out to see how we practise and obviously if we have any problems or troubles we contact them*

and:

> *The supervisor came out, she worked with me, I guess she interviewed me, it wasn't a formal sit down interview.*

Many midwives saw the supervisor as carrying out a purely managerial and particularly disciplinary role:

> *There is no difference in their duties than that of a manager... all she does are management duties.*

> *She just uses it as a disciplinary tool... we only see her if there is a problem.*

This is recognised by some supervisors:

> *If I don't know the midwives well for whom I am a supervisor, sometimes they don't see my role as supervisor any differently from my role as manager and I think that probably is the biggest obstacle.*

Other midwives stressed more strongly that some supervisors were clinicians rather than managers and mentioned the advantages that held:

> *Because she is working with us every day... she knows everyone's practice.*

Yet, the way in which supervisors who are clinically based are deployed clearly affects their supervisory role:

We hardly ever see them... they come in from the community occasionally.

It is difficult... I have been waiting for my review since last April (18 months) but I still haven't had it. The only time she is on the ward doing a shift is if she is rostered onto the ward as a midwife... but then obviously you haven't got time to sit down and take time to discuss issues, it is difficult for her.

However, others felt a balance was achieved:

I think we are lucky here, in that we have both. We have clinicians and managers, so one probably compensates for the other.

Supervisory contacts

The traditional formal often 'annual' interview (although formally planned it does not appear to take place every year) was a common method of supervision as the comments of these midwives illustrate:

We are supposedly having our what do you call it, like a self review... like an annual appraisal.

The last meeting I went to I had to take along sets of notes... and I suppose an audit of my record keeping took place. I also had to show my equipment and that was checked as well and also a general discussion about how I felt about issues within the unit.

However, an 'annual review' did not suit everyone:

Meeting someone once a year is not sufficient and the meeting that you have with that person is highly superficial... that to me isn't ongoing support as it should be.

Each unit studied in this phase of the research had a version of a supervisory checklist or self-review form which facilitated discussions around personal and professional development as well as practice issues. Some units were changing the format in line with the changes they envisaged and anticipated occurring locally with supervision.

Frequency of meetings between supervisors and midwives varied from daily or weekly, especially for those with clinically based supervisors, to once every three years for one midwife:

It must have been about three years ago that I met with her, she came out to supervise my practice.

Every time I see her (either daily or weekly) she asks if 'things are OK with you?', 'is there anything you want to ask me', that sort of thing... she takes more of an interest than other midwives.

An additional method of supervising was that of group supervision. It was viewed in a positive light and valued by those experiencing it:

We used to have a monthly supervision hour... in a group... just talk about what was going on or things that might be relevant like litigation.

Time for supervision

The findings in the first phase revealed that only 22 per cent of supervisors had specific time allowed for supervisory duties. The lack of time allocated to supervision was reiterated in several ways. An acknowledgement was made that more could be done within the framework of supervision but that time constraints restrict supervisory practice:

We are very restricted with the amount of time that we actually devote to supervision.

Supervision could be better but they [the supervisors] *haven't got the time.*

A number of those interviewed felt that supervision was not meeting the needs of midwives and that time pressure generally was an issue:

I think they need more time to speak to an individual – more time for them... meetings now and again to... discuss things that are going on in general.

Other aspects of the role

Acting as a 'sounding board' was one aspect which was commented upon on many occasions, often to 'clarify issues':

It is very important they have got a sounding board, somebody that they can talk to ...

A counselling/support role was also predominant in many supervisors' and supervisees' comments:

... it gives them a chance to off load on me if they find things a bit stressful.

Support was seen to be crucial, particularly in the present climate of rapid change within the service as a whole, in addition to the changing philosophy and working patterns in midwifery care specifically. The needs of the midwife were also seen by some as being a crucial aspect of 'safeguarding the public'; 'it is a support network to protect the public and to protect the midwives'. Others suggested that supporting and enabling the midwife would in turn be a way of protecting the public.

... support them the whole way in making changes.

support... making sure they are not in trouble... supporting them in their practice, being there for advice.

Protecting the midwife was seen as essential. Many midwives were considered to be endeavouring to undertake too much:

They are just going to burn out, we've nearly lost one [midwife]... she was just going overboard... she was just burning herself out.

Some people move a lot faster than others (in terms of change) and the people who are not keeping up I think need a certain amount of support and protection because otherwise you find you are losing some.

Importance of the personal relationship

Setting aside the employed position of the supervisor, many midwives viewed the actual personal relationship as being the important aspect:

It depends on the supervisor and the relationship the midwife has with the supervisor... I find mine quite approachable and I'll go off and discuss everything with her but if you've got, you know, if there's a problem of personalities or problems that a midwife wouldn't approach a supervisor with, then I think it isn't, it's not facilitating properly.

I have quite free access to my supervisor, as and when I need it. I suppose I am quite fortunate... I think if you have a good relationship, that is important.

I see supervisors coming in as a more personal thing now rather than before, they used to be a policing service didn't they and that's not what it's going to be now.

And, as one midwife suggested:

Certainly you need a good attitude towards fellow midwives. This hasn't always been so with some supervisors I have come across. I have seen some quite threatening figures really as supervisors.

Changes in the nature of supervision

Change in the practice of supervision was clearly apparent in all of the case studies. For example, the formal interviews were typically being held 'once a year at the moment, but I know that is changing'.

The historical context and precedent were evident but many saw the transition taking place:

There is still the stigma of the supervisor having a policing type of role in addition to a facilitating mentor type of role.

It's changing, it's in its infancy and I can see that perhaps supervision in three or four years time is going to be different from the way it is now, but it's just starting so I suppose I come from the background where the supervisor was just there if something was, if you had done something wrong or if something wrong had happened but I can see that that is going to be changing.

Historically the supervisors have always been there if clinically you had done something wrong, and I think for midwives to move away from that is going to take a long time, so having a supervisor available clinically for a lot of midwives this is going to be different, but I think it will take time to change.

A vision for the future of supervision was expressed by one midwife:

I think it will be different and maybe with the people I see going on the supervisor courses now, are midwives working with the midwives, you know who are there every day knowing what's going on and what's happening and how you feel and everything... I am looking forward to having a supervisor who is more clinically based.

There was an emphasis on the idea that some midwives themselves had to change their attitudes towards supervision as well as the supervisors in the way they function:

> I can see that it's improving or that it's going to improve. I think that midwives have got to recognise that first.

Raising the profile of supervision not only with midwives but also with the public was considered to be vital:

> I think it has progressed certainly, I think it's much more high profile now and it's being used more effectively and I think all midwives are becoming aware of that. I still don't think the public have much knowledge yet about midwifery supervision and what it can do and I don't think supervisors themselves realise what strength they could use really.

General views on the role

Supervisors' comments regarding their role confirmed many of the responses made in the questionnaire-based survey but were elaborated in some areas. Supervisors clearly valued the role highly although some acknowledged that many supervisors do not understand the powerful role that supervision represents. The overriding opinion, as in the questionnaire survey, was that the principal aim of supervision was to 'protect the public', a role undertaken in a variety of ways. There was clearly tension between actually undertaking the protection of the public role in a monitoring way, and being seen as a disciplinarian, as well as having a role to support the midwife. Some midwives did not hold supervision in very high regard: 'It is more a disciplinary tool than anything else.'

Another way of tackling this monitoring/disciplinarian aspect of the role for some supervisors was that they believed that developing the formative work would reduce the incidence of the normative work. One example would be that the supervisor identified areas in which education about certain practice issues would be valuable to ensure that practice was of a standard required. This was viewed as a means of preventing incidents occurring which could potentially lead to poor practice, which was related to their role of protecting the public.

The differing roles of the supervisors was interesting and varied, some saw the manager supervisor as being distant, 'someone you would see occasionally' and 'only if there is a problem' whereas the clinical supervisor 'was more accessible' for some. Yet others thought that as some clinically based supervisors, particularly if community based, did not understand how the unit worked, then they would only 'call them if we're absolutely desperate'. Ultimately, though, there seemed to be an opinion that a mixture of supervisors who were clinically and managerially based would be the ideal situation:

> *I think you need input from different areas as well because otherwise you get a very biased view and perhaps an unrealistic view sometimes, sometimes you want to change the world and it's not feasible within today's climate.*

Some clear expectations regarding supervision were expressed by midwives:

> *Getting together, meetings and sitting down, seeing what we want, what they want to achieve, generally sort of sitting down and getting feedback from the midwives.*

> *Being a sounding board for us, someone we can discuss practice issues with confidentially, without it being raised as an issue for IPR.*

Overall they felt that there was a change in supervision which was viewed as being positive. In areas where considerable developments had been made, both the midwives and supervisors viewed the transition as beneficial and the move to supporting individuals and yet challenging midwives to develop their practice further was clearly evident:

> *They encourage us to go on courses... which is good... it took a lot of courage to start doing something... and you do look at your practice much more... I think we were a bit complacent.*

> *That is always something that comes up at our, my annual review, you know, something to actually try and do more of, achieve more in practice terms.*

This final statement suggests that supervision can potentially impact on practice, which was an area explored further within the interviews, with particular emphasis on the achievement of specific service targets stated within the Protocol.

Impact of supervision on practice

When exploring whether supervision has an impact on practice a lack of clarity in roles was evident. In terms of whether supervision could directly impact on the targets within the Protocol, both supervisors and midwives deliberated whether it was a management role or a supervisory role.

> *I think I would say I think it's a bit of both management and supervision and a lot of them will probably have a resource implication and an organisational implication as well as obviously training needs and updating.*

> *I have more of a role in my management capacity in the Protocol.*

Midwives themselves were also confused as to whether the individuals were acting in a management capacity or as a supervisor:

> *I know that supervisors were involved in it but they were also managers so I don't know which role they were involved as.*

> *I don't think that is her role as a supervisor, it is a management role.*

Others acknowledged that both management and supervisory functions play a part:

> *It is a bit of both management and supervision although a lot of them will probably have resource and organisational implications as well, which are more management issues.*

Where the supervisor was also the principal manager, the confusion was clearly more evident, yet in many cases the role was seen positively:

> *She understands the needs of the unit as well as the midwifery staff.*

Others would see this dual management/supervisor role as a problem, as supervision can be used as a management tool to implement change.

> *[It is] difficult being the manager of the unit and implementing change but also being the supervisor of others who were against what she wanted for this unit.*

I think it is a bit difficult to mix management with things like that and being supervisor as well because there are all sorts of things that you would turn to the supervisor for help and advice on, which you would have a conflict of ideas with a manager.

Direct or indirect approach

When considering the impact supervision had had on working towards improvements in care, a variety of practices were found. The variation in practice ranged from a direct approach, adopted by some supervisors, to a more discreet and less tangible way of working towards the targets, as these examples illustrate:

We, as supervisors, went through the documents last year, picked out certain aspects in particular to what we are doing and are we achieving all the things that we wanted to do... we then went back to our work places and spoke to the other midwives... so that everyone has an input.

Well I think in looking at what midwives want so that they feel supported, maybe you have a midwife who was very keen to get out into a continuity of care team but perhaps needed some updating in delivery suite or something. Then we would obviously accommodate them there, making sure that the rest of the service is left at a safe level.

It is really like a co-operation you know, that all the midwives need to work towards these influences to change, a supervisor cannot do it on her own but probably the midwives cannot do it on their own either.

During the formal supervisory interviews undertaken with midwives, issues relating to the Protocol in general were discussed.

We talk about it very broadly and specifically within the formal meetings that I have with midwives... I wouldn't have any other time outside of my job as it is at the moment, to do any more.

An alternative view was that changing practice in relation to the targets within the Protocol was an issue for individual midwives.

I would have thought it was the responsibility of the midwife to meet these targets, but if they were stuck they could ask for some assistance or guidance.

In contrast, others suggested that the targets were discussed and addressed from the supervisors' point of view, in both a global view and from more specific notions as these three examples indicate:

By supporting the rationale behind them... we have done talks on them and midwives have done assignments on them and we ask them to bring them back and do a seminar about their assignment.

She [supervisor] *encouraged us and sent us on courses to develop the Baby Friendly Initiative.*

We needed to develop parentcraft so she [supervisor] *helped us go on courses to do that.*

A more indirect approach

Working with clinicians, on a multi-professional basis, and 'setting an example', 'being a role model', offering women choice and acting as an advocate, were clear examples of how the respondents thought supervision could affect practice, with an emphasis given to it being:

... a background way, a subtle way rather than being dictatorial. Leading from behind.

A midwife also acknowledged this purpose of supervision:

She has been supportive of what we are doing, but she hasn't necessarily trail blazed directly, although I think indirectly she has been quite influential.

One midwife in particular felt that support was crucial:

Support enables me to be more confident in my practice.

Support during the change and development of practice was seen to be crucial to success when implementing new schemes and some supervisors saw that as their role.

Some will come with a suggestion... use you as a sounding board... and then you'd support them.

Others felt that actually working with midwives was a crucial way of improving practice:

> *going in and assisting with deliveries, maybe going in and taking the baby and afterwards doing a debriefing, we are keen to do it with the women but don't do it enough with the midwives and maybe we don't say to them enough – that was a really nice delivery ...*

However, others did not feel that supervision had much impact at all:

> *The fact that you have a supervisor of midwives, or if you were a supervisor of midwives, I don't think that is going to affect the work practices or the target achievement.*

Yet, when discussing the role of the supervisor in the professional development of midwives it was clear that many supervisors considered that intervening in establishing and finding ways of meeting the development needs of midwives was a way of impacting on practice.

> *I think they [supervisors] should be guiding midwives through their career, advising them to continue their ongoing education and maybe talk to them about areas they would like to expand their education, in an advisory capacity.*

> *They point me in the right direction, being an older midwife I haven't done as many courses as the younger midwives that are coming in, so that they do point me in the right direction and we discuss things.*

Updating sessions were organised by managers and supervisors alike. Many of the educational issues were identified at supervisory interviews and resulted in educational/developmental activities being organised:

> *We can tell her [supervisor] what we feel we need experience in, (for example, suturing, she got someone to come in and give us a talk).*

Impact on practice in relation to some Protocol targets

The interviews focused on many of the targets set within the Protocol. However, the variety of opinions suggested that it depended on the individual approach of the supervisor and on the interpretation of the role by both parties as to how supervision affects practice and the achievement of the targets. For example, one target within the Protocol was that of continuity of carer, where the named midwife or a small group of known midwives provide midwifery care either in the hospital or in the community. Many of the case study areas have either considered ways of achieving this target or implemented schemes which enhanced or provided this type of care.

Supervision did not appear to have a direct impact on this target. However, there were examples where the support given by supervisors enabled midwives to take practice forward in this direction. Yet, the organisation of alternative methods of work organisation often had resource and manpower implications and was therefore considered more a management issue.

Implementing midwifery led care had been an area of discussion between some supervisors and midwives. In areas where midwifery led care had been implemented the supervisors' role was not entirely clear:

> We have a pilot team starting... supervisors were involved on the working group but I don't know if that was in their role as a manager.

In other areas, whilst trying to implement midwifery led care, supervisors had had to overcome resistance from other professional colleagues. Both the supervisors and managers had a role in overcoming this resistance. The supervisor was instrumental in defining roles and territories and also supporting the midwives during 'battle fatigue'. Both the supervisors and managers were involved in discussing and debating the issues relating to midwifery led care. Although success in this area had not been high, the supervisors had played an advocacy role as well as supporting midwives establishing this method of working and providing a forum to discuss practice issues.

This theme of a combined management and supervisory role, when endeavouring to improve practice and achieve the targets within the Protocol, continued as other areas were discussed. It was often unclear as to whether the supervisor had had a clear direct impact on the targets in question. Often it depended on the particular interests of the supervisor, with breast feeding being one example.

In a few areas the midwives had worked particularly hard on improving and maintaining breast feeding rates (a specific target is stated in the Protocol). In some areas the supervisors had been actively involved, working with groups writing breast feeding policies and addressing the improvement of the uptake and maintenance of breast feeding.

> *I know our supervisor has been actively involved with the breast feeding group... the supervisors did set up workshops on breast feeding.*

As one respondent suggested, the approach taken really depended on the interests of the individual supervisor:

> *She* [supervisor] *is really keen on supporting breast feeding and has worked hard in that area.*

Others were not clear whether the supervisor had a role in this area:

> *I think in general as a midwife you should be promoting breast feeding, obviously, and going around with the views and ideas on how to improve the breast feeding rate but I don't know how they could directly in their role as a supervisor.*

Individual supervisors who had a particular interest in this area and had obviously worked hard achieved an improvement in practice. However, this could be more from their professional interest than a direct supervisory action. Yet, having the additional role as a supervisor may have assisted in channelling information and facilitating educational development in the area and therefore indirectly improving practice.

A more direct application of supervision could be seen in relation to the target regarding women having 'a positive experience of childbirth' (WHPF, 1991). One aspect of this target saw the role of the supervisor as protector of the public, dealing with complaints from women who had had a less than positive experience. However, this could be interpreted as a reactive, rather than a proactive role as supervisors were involved in investigating the complaint.

In terms of supervisors affecting the positive experience of childbirth in a more proactive manner, direct impact was difficult to discern. In some areas supervisors acted as support to midwives concerned about individual clients and any specific practice issues.

Other targets were discussed and the results were similar, in that it depended upon whether changes implemented were a direct result of actions taken by the supervisor or a result of management initiative. Similarly, many did not view the achievement of the targets as a responsibility of the supervisor. However, there was some tentative evidence that supervision had an indirect role in assisting in this area by supporting midwives with the changes occurring to meet women's needs and the implementation of schemes to meet the target areas.

The importance of a relationship

Throughout the data collected it was evident that the individual characteristics of the person appointed as a supervisor enabled a positive supervisory role. The relationship they created and established with supervisees seemed to have a significant impact on improving practice. However, organisational factors, for example location and supervision ratios, will impact on the making and maintenance of good relationships. For example, a number of midwives had suggested that they sought advice from supervisors, or used them as a 'sounding board' to discuss ideas or reflect on practice issues. To undertake this aspect of supervision, the relationship had to be such that the supervisor could express her views without causing offence:

> [It is] *being able to say, well you are going to be absolutely exhausted if you do that – you are really going to wear yourself out – and actually get them to see the problem, not actually being critical because you don't want to dampen down their initiative and enthusiasm.*

Similarly, midwives expressed a view that they would approach their supervisors for anything, and therefore viewed their relationship as a safe environment to discuss issues:

> *... she is there for me and I always feel free to pick up a phone at any time if I need to discuss something.*

When describing the effectiveness of supervision one midwife said:

> *It needs to grow out of the sense of relationship and trust and friendship and from that comes security, and from that grows the ability to share more openly with each other, and then learn from each other.*

Similarly, others focused on the relationship side of supervision and stressed that it was of paramount importance:

> *I think* [the effectiveness of supervision] *is more dependent on personality.*

> *I do think it depends on the relationship – perhaps some of the midwives who haven't known her so long don't find it so easy to use her for support.*

> *Sometimes they want to look at my equipment and sometimes they don't. It's much more a question of getting to know each other.*

The development of such a relationship appears to enable the supervisor to have an understanding and knowledge of each midwife's strengths and weaknesses, in terms of both the individual's practice and professional development. For many, this relationship did not seem to depend on whether the supervisor was employed as a manager or as a clinician. The relationship would appear to be more dependent on the individual characteristics of the person. However, a number of supervisors expressed concern regarding the occasions when an individual wished to discuss particular issues with their supervisor, but were inhibited because of the supervisor's additional managerial role and the implications that might have. Recognition was, however, given to managers who were seen to be potentially supportive in different ways, by representing midwives in different circles. For example:

> [it is] *about supporting midwives... they get so frustrated at times... it's representing them as well at directorate level.*

> [For the] *protection of the midwife and midwifery, you will always need those ones that are communicating with other professionals on a wider front... you need those in a top notch position, leadership position... although I think sometimes supervisors are hampered by their management roles, that often overtakes them in their supervisory roles.*

> *Because of her senior position she would be influential in other areas.*

For midwives where an effective relationship was not seen to be established, the supervisory role was viewed purely as a monitoring tool and the true potential of the role was inhibited. In this type of situation midwives were reluctant to call their supervisor in an emergency situation, and also inhibited from approaching the supervisor to discuss and debate issues, or seeking their support and advice in taking practice forward:

There is no point really [in approaching the supervisor]. *I would rather talk to my colleague than her.*

I don't find her supportive at all. You only ever see her if there is a problem.

No, I don't think supervision is effective... I don't find I can talk to her... she just checks my bags and watches my practice.

The relationship between supervisor and supervisee may also be affected by the interpretation of the role of supervision by the supervisors themselves and their reason for being a supervisor. The motivation of the supervisor also affects the relationship:

She's OK as a person but I don't think she is effective at supervision.

Some people are driven by power and I think if people are going to apply for a supervisor's post seeing it as a position of power, I can see that there would be a breakdown in relationships and it's not going to work because people aren't going to relate to that person and they have to feel that they can go to someone who's going to relate to them on the same level as them and be non-judgmental and be there to support, but equally they have to offer constructive criticism and there are some people that are very good at that and able to do it effectively and there are some people that aren't at all suitable for the post, so I suppose it's going to be down to personalities.

She just uses supervision as a disciplining tool.

Discussion

The individual characteristics of the supervisor, and the way the supervisor interprets and acts out the role of supervision have an impact on whether supervision is viewed positively by midwives and has an affect on their practice. Certainly one could argue that supervision is fulfilling the role of protector of the public and that of maintaining standards in the monitoring side of supervision. Yet, often the supervisor is reacting to incidents as they occur rather than protecting the public from potential harm from bad practice by identifying possible problems before they occur.

However, there was evidence that the attitude towards and the enactment of supervision was changing. The punitive role was being replaced with a more challenging and supportive role similar to the model described by Daloz (1986). With this model, adequate support and challenge can be seen to develop the individual in a positive direction and hence potentially take practice forward. An imbalance between support and challenge can have the opposite effect and could have detrimental effects by either confirming an individual's ability/practice and causing stagnation in practice development or by over-challenging an individual to the point of regression or inability to perform at all. Certainly within this study there was evidence that where midwives had been encouraged to attend courses and were supported through the duration they had benefited both personally and professionally. This apparently new direction of supervision was certainly valued by those who had experienced it.

Conclusions

Some of the findings may appear stark. In particular, it is striking that, after ninety-five years of statutory supervision, there is little clear evidence within the literature that supervision improves the quality of care given to women using the maternity services. However, in terms of self-regulation, supervision has a clear remit and the monitoring side of the role ensures that safe standards of care are maintained. In the light of clinical governance the supervision of midwives would appear to fulfil many of the issues being discussed at present within other organisations as a means of self-regulation.

However, the clear move from a purely monitoring and direct quality control definition of the supervisor's role, to one in which the supervisor attempts to influence practice indirectly by education and development has implications for the way in which supervision is organised. In particular, it raises a question over the two roles (plus in many cases a third, management, role) remaining in the hands of one person. This is certainly a notion discussed by the Association of Radical Midwives

(1994) in terms of splitting the role of monitoring from that of support, counselling and development.

There is a good case for arguing that the supervision ratio, even when within the regulatory guidance (UKCC, 1998), is too large for supervision to be effective. This is particularly pertinent given the broad way in which many supervisors interpret their role in practice and the importance midwives attached to the development of a personal relationship.

Midwifery and supervisory practice have been changing markedly in recent years. Reorganisations of health care provision, the introduction of new models of midwifery care, the concept of woman-centred care, the increasing number of clinicians who are supervisors, the introduction of clinical supervision in nursing and the expansion in the number of supervisors all contribute to a situation in which the researchers were standing on shifting sand. The shift is continuing. Since the study was completed the supervisor–midwife ratio has improved dramatically, from 1:31 to 1:17 (personal communication) and more clinicians have been appointed as supervisors including those employed at F grade.

The study has provided for the first time a reasonably clear picture of what is happening with midwifery supervision in Wales. It has provided a benchmark, a snapshot at one point in time, with which later results can be compared. The results have also provoked further questions, which could be the subject of more structured and focused research.

The question of whether supervision improves practice is more fundamental. From the data collected within this research project it was difficult to discern a clear direct relationship between supervision and practice although there is tentative evidence that there is an indirect relationship. If the supervisory role becomes more challenging and supportive this relationship may become more clearly apparent in the future. Similarly, the coming of audit and of the Clinical Effectiveness Initiative gives us a chance to gather new evidence.

Survey of lead supervisors in Wales

The aim of this part of the study was to explore in detail the role and responsibilities of the lead supervisors. The 1995 Health Authorities Act had resulted in a recent restructuring of the local supervising authority

(LSA). Therefore, we looked at the role before and after the Act to assess the impact on the lead supervisor.

Research methods

The project team sought to elicit data from the lead supervisors themselves, in order to interpret their concepts of the role and explore the activities undertaken by the lead supervisors. The initial data were collected by telephone interviews. Lead supervisors in Wales during 1995 and 1996 (n=10) were invited to participate.

Nine months after the interviews took place, and after the implementation of the reorganisation created by the Health Authorities Act, a focus group was held to discuss the findings from the interviews. This enabled a further discussion to take place regarding the role of the lead supervisor, in addition to the identification and consideration of any changes that may have occurred as a result of the reorganisation.

Results

The appointment as a lead supervisor and time in post

There was considerable variety in the way in which the lead supervisors had been appointed originally. A number had been appointed by virtue of their position as manager of the maternity services in that particular area, for example '… it went with the post that I now hold.' Others had been invited to apply for the position with other colleagues. At the time of the interviews the lead supervisors had been in post varying periods of time ranging from ten months to ten years.

As a result of the changes brought about by the implementation of the Health Authorities Act 1995, two of the group had been invited to reapply for the position as lead supervisor and had been reappointed. Others continued with their current appointment although in one case an additional post was created to facilitate the appropriate representation of a large geographical area.

Training

Training for the post was a significant theme. None of the participants had had any preparation to undertake the role of lead supervisor. A common experience was, 'my training was a 15 minute chat'. Some viewed the position as 'a role you grow into' and many had been dependent on their relationship with the Chief Administrative Nursing Officer (CANO) for guidance on how to fulfil their role. There was unanimous agreement that training would be useful.

I didn't have any official training but I did have a lot of guidance and support in the first year.

It depends on your previous experience, but some training would have been useful, even just a job description would have helped.

Establishing the role of the lead supervisor

The range of activities of the lead supervisor were based upon the UKCC guidance (UKCC, 1993 and 1998) with additional aspects to the role influenced by the CANO and the particular needs of an area:

It depends on the area, if there are particular problems I would visit more frequently and devise an action plan with the unit.

However, there would appear to be the potential of developing the role further in the new health authorities. With the coming of the Act, many of those interviewed indicated that there was an opportunity to raise the profile of supervision, both at authority and at trust level. Some felt that the lead supervisor role could become a full-time one in order to develop the role further and to allow other issues such as additional work with the commissioning teams to be addressed. The changes were generally viewed as an exciting opportunity. As one respondent suggested:

Supervision of midwifery was now on many agendas and the profile of supervision and the statutory function had been raised.

Many lead supervisors had used reorganisation as an opportunity to ensure that midwifery services 'had a voice' in many more circles and 'ensured that there was provision of unbiased information to purchasers, trusts and educational institutions'.

The activities of a lead supervisor, as reported by those interviewed, were diverse. The main roles identified were that of coordinating the statutory requirements, setting standards and influencing policy and practice by being an advocate for the midwifery profession at various management levels.

The potential of the role

An important theme was the way in which the respondents viewed the role itself and the potential of the role. All the lead supervisors who were interviewed considered the role to be valuable and essential but many also viewed the role as 'potentially powerful', a view supported by the responsible officers in England (Nobles, 1996).

This potential often took the form of power to influence decision making to advance the status of the midwifery profession. Certainly respondents felt that with the changes in the health services as a whole, the impact of the lead supervisor at health authority level has the potential to be extremely beneficial for the women using the services.

If the trust are not willing to discuss or consider issues which affect the safety of mothers and babies then the lead supervisor can go to the health authority to address the same.

The role of the lead supervisor was seen as being both vital and potentially powerful in ensuring that standards within trusts were maintained and in representing midwifery within the trusts at health authority level.

Other aspects of lead supervision, where there was potential for development, included the promotion of the clinical effectiveness agenda and the encouragement of evidence-based care, at both health authority and trust level. Some of those interviewed referred specifically to the introduction of risk management into the work of the lead supervisor, in addition to risk management beginning to feature in midwifery supervision generally.

Discussion regarding the lead supervisors

The function of the lead supervisor, as characterised and practised by the lead supervisors themselves, is a long way from that of 'monitor of standards' as envisaged in statute and regulatory guidance. It has evolved into a much broader and more complex role. In their view the potential of the role to influence was significant. They appeared to naturally envisage the role as one of leadership, the leading professional, since the power to influence has been generally accepted for some time as a key characteristic of leaders (French and Raven, 1968).

The lead supervisors acted out their power to influence in a number of ways, for example within their managerial responsibilities they can be seen to act as a networker, monitor of standards, policy adviser and formulator and decision influencer. Through these activities they saw themselves as advocates for the profession with a responsibility for giving it a voice which will be heard. For the midwifery profession, the case for this role is a strong one; it would be difficult to argue against it.

Given this breadth, complexity and importance, the lack of preparation for and training in the role and the varied way in which the lead supervisors are appointed is surprising but may be due to the rapidly evolving nature of the role. The lack of specification of duties and the amount of time the lead supervisors are expected to allocate to them, and the lack of clarity in the way in which remuneration is made are similarly surprising but also explainable. The overall impression is that organisational structures and processes are not keeping pace with a rapidly evolving role. The task for those creating that organisational infrastructure is to ensure that it does not inappropriately constrain the development of the lead supervisor's role. The reorganisation following the Health Authorities Act 1995 has possibly presented a useful opportunity.

Glossary

The model of supervision described by Proctor (1986) has three interactive functions.

Normative: described by Proctor as the managerial and quality control functions of supervision. These functions could include monitoring of practice, dealing with complaints, checking drugs and other direct, if negative, methods of trying to ensure a high quality of practice and to ensure the safety of mother, baby and the public.

Formative: described by Proctor as the educative function of supervision. These functions could include discussion, encouragement, arranging courses and other positive, if indirect, methods of trying to ensure a high quality of practice and to ensure the safety of mother, baby and the public.

Restorative: described by Proctor as the support and counselling functions of supervision. These functions are intended to help midwives themselves to handle stressful situations.

References

Association of Radical Midwives (1994). 'Supervision working party: first draft proposals for future midwifery supervision'. *Midwifery Matters*, No. 60, pp. 26-27.

Daloz, L.A. (1986). *Effective Teaching and Mentoring: Realising the Transformational Power of Adult Learning Experiences*. London: Jossey-Bass.

Flint, C. (1985). 'Trouble and strife'. *Nursing Times*, Vol. 81, No. 45, p. 22.

French, J.R., Raven, B. (1968). 'The bases of social power'. In: Cartwright, D., Zander, A.F. (eds) *Group Dynamics: research and theory*. London: Harper and Rowe.

Kargar, I. (1993). 'Whither supervision?' *Nursing Times,* Vol. 89, No. 40, p. 22.

Kirkham, M. (1995). 'History of midwifery supervision'. In: Association of Radical Midwives. *Super-Vision. Consensus Conference Proceedings*. Hale: Books for Midwives Press.

Leap, N., Hunter, B. (1993). *The Midwife's Tale*. London: Scarlet Press.

Mayes, G. (1995). *Supervisors Of Midwives – How can we Facilitate Change? The challenge of change to meet the challenge of 'Changing Childbirth'*: Midwifery Educational Resource Pack: Section 5:33-42. London: ENB.

Nobles, W. (1996). Letter re 'UKCC statement on practice nurses.' *British Journal of Midwifery* Vol. 4, No. 9, p. 457.

Proctor, B. (1986). 'Supervision: a co-operative in accountability.' In: Marken, M., Payne, M. (eds) *Enabling and Ensuring*. Leicester National Youth Bureau and Council for Education and Training in Youth and Community Work.

UKCC (1993) *Midwives Rules*. London: UKCC.

UKCC (1998) *Midwives Rules and Code of Practice*. London: UKCC.

Walton, I. (1995). 'Conflicts in supervision of midwives.' In: Association of Radical Midwives. *Super-Vision. Consensus Conference Proceedings*. Hale: Books for Midwives Press.

WHPF (Welsh Health Planning Forum) (1991). *Protocol for Investment in Health Gain: Maternal and Early Child Health*. Welsh Office: Cardiff.

The next three chapters are derived from a study of supervision in England, commissioned jointly by the ENB and UKCC. It is published in full by the ENB (Stapleton, Duerden and Kirkham 1998). Six sites in England were studied: five very different National Health Service sites and one consisting of non-NHS midwives working in independent practice or privately employed. Ethics Committee approval was gained in all areas.

Jean Duerden

Audit of Supervision of Midwives
England 1996-7

RESEARCH AND AUDIT

Having already audited the supervision of midwives in the North West Health Region in 1994-1995 (Duerden, 1995), when I was invited to join the research team commissioned by the ENB and the UKCC to evaluate the impact of the supervision of midwives on professional practice, it seemed logical to repeat the work done in the North West on the six chosen sites in England. There was, in addition, a golden opportunity to introduce to the study the aspects of the audit which I would have loved to change during the North West Project which, with hindsight, would have helped the original study, though by the time the need for these amendments had become apparent, it was too far into that study to take remedial action.

The new study produced the ENB report *Evaluation of the Impact of the Supervision of Midwives on Professional Practice and the Quality of Midwifery Care* (Stapleton et al, 1998). The report contains all the statistical evidence in full from the study.

As might be expected, halfway into the English study new issues had arisen which would have been useful if included. In particular, I would have liked to see confidentiality included, as this was raised so many times by midwives during the in-depth interviews by the research midwife.

The earlier study identified two groups of midwives who appeared to have particular problems with determining their eligibility to practise as midwives. These were either midwives working in neonatal units or midwife teachers/lecturers, each with their own anxieties regarding their practice. It seemed to be appropriate, therefore, to separate them out from the study and to ask questions pertinent to that issue. As the first audit had proved successful, and had prtovided a good picture of the supervisory service, no other amendments were made.

The terms of reference in the North West study were to undertake a systematic and independent examination of supervision of midwives, to examine the current local guidelines for supervision, to determine whether supervisory activities and related outcomes comply with current guidelines and to determine whether the arrangements for and practice of supervision of midwives are consistent. It therefore remained an appropriate tool for this study, with the North West audit providing a comparison for the new research.

The audit

For the England study fewer midwives were interviewed, in total 159 midwives on six sites, plus 11 midwives working in neonatal units on three of the sites. In addition, 27 supervisors and 15 midwife teachers were also interviewed across five sites. There were no refusals to be audited by midwives or supervisors. As few as four, and as many as 19, midwives and from one to four supervisors were interviewed in one day.

In contrast with the earlier audit, this study did not focus on one geographical area, but reached five very different parts of the country, from north to south. The length of visit to each site varied, depending on the number and size of the maternity units and the geographic location. Peripheral units were usually audited in half a day, with a minimum of a full day required for each district hospital. On the two sites where there were no peripheral units involved, visits over two consecutive days were made to interview a larger number of midwives. An attempt was made to interview all the supervisors of midwives and as many of the midwives on duty who could be seen within the time available.

All midwife teachers with an academic input into each site were included in the audit. Wherever midwives worked in neonatal units, as many as possible were included. There were no midwives working in neonatal units at sites one, five and six. This appears to be common practice now: staff who are registered midwives as well as registered nurses are no longer encouraged to notify their intention to practise as a midwife, as the work they undertake in high dependency units is not considered midwifery practice.

In addition to individual supervisor interviews, a collective interview took place with all the supervisors to look at policies and procedures for supervision across the site. Despite the fact that several peripheral units were in separate trusts, as on site two, there was a sharing between the supervisors with regular meetings, a shared on-call rota and shared philosophies.

The changed midwifery environment

It soon became apparent that the midwifery environment had changed since the North West audit. At that time, I had been aware, from both midwives and supervisors of midwives, of a sense of excitement and challenge from the empowerment offered by *Changing Childbirth* (DoH, 1993). Midwives looked forward to being able to practise as respected, autonomous practitioners. Unfortunately, during this later audit, the climate had changed to one of uncertainty. It appeared that the midwives had acquired completely different agendas, with a change from empowerment and challenge to insecurity and bewilderment. The midwives reported seeing their managers, often supervisors of midwives, as vulnerable, and persistently having to 'kow-tow to trust management' (Duerden, 1997). One midwife in the study said:

> *There is a marked conflict of roles between supervisors and managers within this hospital. Recently in this unit the care of women has been compromised and the supervisor has not been able to take action to ensure safe practice because of management restrictions on staffing and funding.* (G grade site four)

With the imposed pared budgets, proposed developments had been deferred, as funding for pilot projects had come to an end and some *Changing Childbirth* schemes withdrawn. Some managers in one of the units had been asked to 'clear their desks' at short notice and the midwives were concerned that it would next be the turn of their own manager. Midwife managers, who are usually also supervisors of midwives, were no longer perceived as having sufficient clout to make management changes as they were no longer part of the trust decision making network.

> *Our dissatisfaction is out of the supervisor's hands, but she provides someone for us to give vent to our feelings to.* (Midwife site 3)

The supervisors

Over 50 per cent of supervisors are now clinically based and many are E and F grades (Thomas and Mayes, 1996) but in the England study no supervisor interviewed was less than a G grade. Not all were managers, but the majority had some management responsibilities; in fact only five of the supervisors interviewed were employed as midwives without a management title. It was inevitable, therefore, that there was confusion between the supervision and management roles, especially if the incumbent was unable clearly to define her roles to the midwives she supervised. For some it was a real problem:

When managers are supervisors you can understand why some midwives resent supervision. (Midwife site two)

The supervisors in this unit are managers, and I believe there is a great conflict of interest. I feel supervisors should not be managers. (Midwife site three)

It wasn't just the midwives who had the problem; 19 per cent of the supervisors who were also managers said they had difficulty separating their role as manager from that as supervisor, and 26 per cent felt they did sometimes. However, one of the supervisors on site four offered an interesting comment:

I think a good manager is automatically a good supervisor. You can't be one without the other.

The conflict between supervision and management is not inevitable. When acting in either capacity, the objectives are clear and separately defined. If there is a critical incident to be investigated, one person cannot act as manager and supervisor, as the former is acting on behalf of the trust, and the latter as advocate for the midwife with responsibility to the LSA.

The supervisors were predominantly managers, but a clinical specialist, a lecturer practitioner and a midwife teacher were also interviewed as well as clinically based midwives. Fewer than 20 per cent of the supervisor population interviewed were clinically based, in contrast to current ENB statistics.

Midwife teachers as supervisors

There is divided opinion as to the appropriateness of a midwife teacher undertaking the role of supervisor of midwives. It is acknowledged that the isolation of academic establishments can hinder the supervisor-supervisee relationship, but those teachers who spend a lot of time in the clinical placement area may have greater contact with midwives than the midwifery manager supervisor. As professional development of midwives is a key responsibility for the supervisor, a midwife teacher can play an important role in encouraging that development.

The midwife teacher and lecturer-practitioner supervisors interviewed shared the on-call duties with colleague supervisors and carried similar case-loads of midwives. This arrangement was well accepted, indeed, one of the most respected and popular supervisors in this study, and probably the most admired by the midwives on that site, held the role of lecturer-practitioner, which position included some management responsibility.

The lecturer-practitioner is probably the most ideally placed to be a supervisor and there is an increasing trend for midwives holding this post to become supervisors. In the North West study, one of the midwife teacher supervisors supervised her colleagues in the university but did not carry a case-load of midwives in the maternity unit where she had clinical links. This was not well received by colleagues, as they felt they were already supervised from an academic aspect by the approved midwife teacher, and a university based supervisor of midwives would not be able to assess the practice needs of those she supervised. In this later study, the midwife- teacher supervisors also supervised their teacher colleagues, but in addition to the midwives they supervised at their clinical link sites.

Length of appointment as a supervisor

The time since appointment as a supervisor of those interviewed varied from six months to 15 years, with an interesting contrast from site to site. On one site all the supervisors were well-established and on another the supervisors were all relatively newly-qualified. The latter proved particularly interesting as they were providing a new model of supervision, far removed from the traditional model that many of us recall from the seventies. They were very excited about the new developments and invited the research team to the unit to demonstrate the changes they had made. Quite conversely, what we found were midwives who were very dissatisfied with supervision. They had long and painful memories of their treatment by supervisors in the past. Unfortunately, this same unit was going through huge management changes which over-rode all the initiatives that the supervisors were trying to introduce. The new supportive model of supervision could not be recognised in a management climate which viewed every complaint as midwife error which needed disciplinary action through management, with a complete disregard for supervision.

In the unit where the supervisors were longer established and supervision had a well-respected (although traditional) style, incidents were dealt with through supervision, although it was sometimes considered a punitive approach by those who knew of it by hearsay rather than personal experience.

Supervisory policies and procedures

The sites contained differing numbers of trusts, with a total of 12 maternity units within the five different sites where supervisors were interviewed. At some of the sites, supervision was carried out collaboratively with shared policies and procedures, including on-call, across the units, even though one of the sites included separately managed and supervised units.

The majority of midwives in the study were offered cross-supervision, i.e. midwives were supervised by a supervisor who was not their manager. This was not possible in the several small rural units where the only supervisor was also the manager.

Within the units studied, the ratio of midwives to supervisors varied from 15:1 to 51:1, with the average ratio per site varying from 23:1 to 33:1. In 1999 there is an overall ratio of 23 midwives per supervisor in England (Mayes 1999, personal communication) and in most LSAs there is a general desire to reduce their ratios, with the target ratio in Yorkshire being 15 midwives per supervisor.

It must be noted, however, that in the trust where, at the time, 50 midwives were allocated to each of the two supervisors, the supervisors in this trust were much respected and supervision more valued than on the other sites which had far smaller ratios. I am glad to be able to report that this ratio has since reduced dramatically, with the appointment of several more supervisors who have adopted the same model of supervision demonstrated in the unit at the time of the audit.

This audit demonstrated a move away from supervising midwives in particular areas, and only one supervisor predominantly supervised community midwives. This proportion of supervisors with evenly mixed case-loads was greater than that of the North West audit, emphasising the shift.

Various systems of allocation were modelled across the sites, from random to alphabetical allocation; whatever system is adopted each has its own advantages and disadvantages and all supervisors should make themselves available to all midwives within the local team (ENB, 1997).

The audit interviewees generally supported not being supervised by their own manager and many of those who were still supervised by their manager were not happy. One midwife in particular did not like working with her supervisor:

> *We are somehow too near to her. In some ways, it is an advantage to have her here, being accessible, but working with her all the time gives the impression that she is out to find fault, yet criticism is often unjustified and therefore makes me lose confidence in what I am doing. It suggests a rigid type of practice and I feel I get put down if I don't comply.* (Community midwife site two)

The hospital midwives with supervisors who were community midwives were not always happy though. As always, what suits one does not necessarily suit another:

> *I was surprised to be allocated a community midwife, when I have more contact with the supervisors in the hospital. I would like to have more contact with my supervisor.* (Midwife site three)

Supervision of supervisors

The supervisors on one site were supervised by their LSA responsible midwifery officer who carried out an annual supervisory review with each supervisor. Two heads of midwifery preferred to be supervised by colleagues from neighbouring trusts, some were supervised by their peer supervisors or by their head of midwifery, but many were not themselves supervised. It is clear from the recent research into clinical supervision that supervisors have their own needs which should be addressed by supervision for themselves (Butterworth et al, 1992). Similarly, if midwives are expected to value their supervision, then surely it is crucial that supervisors value their own supervision. None of us are above needing to be supervised or having our own practice or professional development needs identified.

Meeting with the LSA responsible officer

As the audit commenced, some local supervising authorities were in a state of flux, as the Health Authorities Act of 1995 was being implemented and the health regions devolved many of their responsibilities, including the statutory responsibility for the supervision of midwives, to health authority level. This meant that each health authority became a local supervising authority, increasing the number of LSAs from 8 to 100. This large number of LSAs meant that consortia had to be formed and an LSA responsible midwifery officer appointed to each consortium. This process was slower in some consortia than others, so at the time of the audit on site one there had not been an appointment and the former link supervisors were continuing with their role as a stopgap. Despite this caretaker arrangement, there were regular LSA meetings and the responsible officers met regularly with the supervisors within every other area audited. This was accomplished by visits to the units and by collective regional meetings with all the supervisors.

All LSA responsible officers are now practising midwives and the opportunities for contact have increased, since their time is allocated for the LSA role, rather than shared with the regional nurse role. The regular LSA meeting provided contact with other supervisors on a fairly regular and frequent basis for the majority of supervisors in the study, with 55 per cent meeting every three months and 89 per cent meeting every six months. This was much more contact than was reported in the North West.

Link supervisors

Following the changes arising from the 1995 Health Authorities Act, there seemed to have been a change in the role of the link supervisor. As all the LSA responsible officers were now midwives, it appeared that some of the officers did not feel it appropriate to use link supervisors. At the time of the audit, when the consortium containing site one was in the process of appointing their first midwife LSA responsible officer, the link supervisors were still well-known and considered relevant to the supervisors at the time of the study.

At site two, the supervisors were uncertain as to who their LSA responsible officer was, as this had been a very recent appointment, although the link supervisor was known and, indeed, had been called in to interview prospective supervisors. Because of the recent changes, it became apparent that there was confusion as to whether or not the link supervisors were still carrying out that role. I later learned from the relevant LSA responsible officers that there were no longer any link supervisors in those regions. In many consortia, it had become common practice for link supervision to cease when a midwife LSA responsible officer had been appointed. The head of midwifery at site five spoke of a link supervisor, but she had no contact with her. This does not mean that there are no longer any link supervisors in England: they exist in several consortia.

Advice on supervision

All the supervisors in the study were questioned on the sources they used for advice and support in their supervisory role: they inevitably used more than one, with the most common being a colleague supervisor. The proportion of supervisors who referred to a colleague was the same as in the North West audit, but a far greater proportion sought advice from the LSA officer. One must assume that having a midwife in the LSA role has brought about this change.

Advice was sought regularly by most of the supervisors but, interestingly, the average period since the last time advice had been sought was the same for the longest serving supervisors as it was for the most recently appointed.

The wider role of the supervisor

Some supervisors had a wider role than simply providing supervision to the midwives on their case-load. Some provided expert advice to outside agencies, but this is an individual arrangement, which some supervisors feel more confident about taking on than others, and carries a large time commitment. Most supervisors said that, as supervisors, they contributed to trust policies, planned schemes which empowered midwives and enabled midwives to prepare for new roles.

Risk management is another of the wider roles that had been taken on by the supervisors. At five of the ten trusts offering maternity services on sites one to five, the supervisors believed they used supervision as a risk management tool and provided many examples of how this was achieved. These examples included providing support and ensuring safe cover at a GP unit; ensuring two midwives attended each home birth; supporting midwives at water births; identifying skills needs at supervisory reviews and offering appropriate, professional update or supervised practice; highlighting the need for stress management; having an incident reporting mechanism; holding lunchtime meetings for case discussion and reflection; using critical incident packages; considering the role of the supervisor in investigation procedures; passing on issues from complaints or critical incidents to the relevant supervisor to see the midwife concerned; instigating practice alerts when at supervisors' meetings issues of good or bad practice were identified; and regular record keeping audits.

One might consider some of these strategies as reactive when risk management should be a proactive endeavour with the risks identified before the incident happens; however, many of these ideas are sufficiently enterprising to be welcomed into the supervisory arena. Supervisors try to sell supervision effectively as a risk management tool to health authorities and trusts; using such initiatives may prevent having to pick up too many complaints or investigate too many critical or clinical incidents.

Methods of supervision of midwives' practice

Monitoring record keeping was seen by the supervisors interviewed in the audit as a key function of the supervisor. They believed that feedback from mothers, including meeting women in clinical practice or on ward visits, was a useful supervisory tool, feedback from staff being equally important. The latter did not necessarily mean midwives reporting on the practice of a colleague, but often on the vulnerable situation on a ward or delivery suite where the staffing levels were too low or the skill-mix was inappropriate. These issues were also highlighted by the supervisors' visits to the wards and observation of clinical practice. Some of the clinically based supervisors felt it was difficult to get an overall view of the service; they felt they had a perspective only on their own work area.

Planned observation of practice was rarely used at the audit sites and remained unique to the community. It was only carried out routinely by six of the supervisors interviewed, fewer than in the North West audit, which suggests that there is a continuing trend to move away from this type of monitoring of practice. One needs to consider, though, if there is still time in the busy supervisor's day to undertake such time-consuming duties.

Midwives themselves were not happy with the concept of supervised visits:

I think direct supervision in the community is a false situation, but it is good to have the opportunity to discuss practice and equipment. I resented supervision when it was first introduced properly, but now it is valued. (Midwife site one)

Preparation of supervisors

During the North West audit, it became evident that the new training of supervisors, using the distance learning pack, facilitated by local universities, had been well received. Seventy-eight per cent of the North West supervisors had been prepared in this way, but only just over half of the supervisors in the England study had been so prepared.

This was a surprise, as the numbers undertaking the preparation course are increasing annually and the English National Board have struggled to accommodate the growing demand. This meant that on the five sites there were fewer supervisors who trained in the last five years compared with the national figure.

When the supervisors were asked if they felt their training had adequately prepared them for their role as a supervisor, as in the North West audit, without exception, those who had been prepared by induction at the English National Board felt they had been inadequately prepared to be a supervisor. Of those who used the open learning pack just two supervisors felt that, even with the new programme, they were still not ready for their role.

The distance learning programme has gone from strength to strength, especially with the introduction of a revised pack. Since the audit many more midwives on the five sites have been prepared as supervisors.

Selection of supervisors

The subject of selection was a point of much debate, both within the audit as well as within the in-depth study. All those interviewed in the audit were asked how they felt supervisors should be selected. Many of the midwives chose two methods of selection. They wanted an election by midwives, supported by selection by interview. Almost half of the teachers would have liked to see midwives being nominated by a supervisor and then the midwives having an opportunity to vote for one of the nominees.

Some other suggestions for selection were made which included self-nomination, open advertisement, peer selection, assessment by an outside body, midwife nomination and selection by midwives from those nominated.

Following the new LSA arrangements, the selection procedure for appointment as a supervisor has improved enormously. My own personal experience of appointment as a supervisor was starting my new post as a midwifery manager one day and receiving a letter of appointment as a supervisor of midwives from the LSA officer, also the regional nurse, the following day.

Now the LSA officer is involved in the selection of all prospective supervisors, involving an interview which includes some academic assessment for ability to complete the preparation course, as well as for determining whether the candidate has suitable qualities to be a supervisor. Self- or peer-nomination is encouraged (ENB, 1996). Election by midwives has been introduced into at least one LSA. This would have been welcomed by midwives in the study:

> *It is important that midwives nominate colleagues rather than it being a decision from the top.* (Midwife site two)

> *Supervisors should be elected midwives with good clinical experience. This democracy would mean that approachable, well qualified midwives will be supervisors.* (Midwife site five)

Choice of supervisor

Midwives in the study were very keen to be able to choose their own supervisor. Many did recognise, however, that this could have disadvantages if everyone were to pick the most popular supervisor, especially if she was popular for the wrong reasons. A good system is to invite midwives to choose three from the list of supervisors whom they would be happy to have as their named supervisor of midwives. This allows choice on both sides, so the supervisor can also choose who she would be content to supervise. Currently the only recommendation (ENB, 1997) is that midwives should be able to change their allocated supervisor if they are unhappy with their supervisory arrangement. The majority of midwives knew they could do this, but not all felt confident in so doing for fear of offending the supervisor concerned.

Midwives in the study

Despite F grade supposedly being the minimum grade for a midwife (EL(95) 77 NHSE 1995), there was no noticeable increase in the number of F grades available for interview since the North West study, although there was a slight shift in that direction. G grades were fewer proportionately, more marked on some sites than others. Trust grades (not Whitley scales) had been introduced on site four.

The majority of the midwives interviewed worked either in hospital or in the community, distinctly separate areas of work, although compared with the North West audit, there was evidence of more team structures and more moves towards an integrated midwifery service, though this only involved 11 per cent of those interviewed.

Access to a supervisor

Twenty-four hour access to a supervisor was available in every trust, with many supervisors carrying either a pager or a mobile phone. Some supervisors did not have such facilities which meant they had to stay by the phone at home if they were on the on-call rota.

Most midwives felt they always had access to a supervisor. For the independent midwives, access was not always so straightforward and some of them had experienced difficulty in making that contact. One midwife from a neonatal unit felt that the supervisors were inaccessible to the neonatal staff and that she would have difficulty contacting a supervisor out-of-hours, probably through lack of knowledge of the on-call system.

Supervisory contact

It was rare to find a midwife who could not identify her supervisor and the five who could not were, without exception, newly qualified or newly appointed. The majority of midwives interviewed had met with their supervisor, some more recently than others, but for the majority within the last six months. The audit demonstrated that midwives approached their supervisor for reasons other than their supervisory review and for a fifth of those interviewed their most recent contact had been for them to seek professional advice from their supervisor. When midwives were asked when they last sought this advice, it was remarkable how many said they had already been to see her that day to ask for advice, demonstrating that midwives are voluntarily going to their supervisors for help.

Only 13 per cent of the midwives interviewed had never sought advice from their supervisor. This was a big improvement on the North West study where 24 per cent had not done so.

Notifications of intention to practise

The administration of notifications of intention to practise held a particular fascination for me. The UKCC form clearly indicates that the supervisor of midwives should receive the notification of intention to practise, but traditionally these have been placed in envelopes on wards for later collection and collation or have been taken to the maternity secretary's office. When the notifications were not pre-printed, I have personal memories of such a secretary standing over me whilst I completed my form, more or less telling me what to put and where. I also recall one maternity unit in the North West study where each midwife had to make an appointment to see her supervisor and complete her notification in her presence. For many of the midwives this meeting was considered the supervisory review. In fact, they referred to the supervisory reviews in that unit as 'notifying intention to practise'.

In this study, the notifications were collated, but not necessarily received, by supervisors in all but one trust. Here, the midwifery manager and maternity secretary took on the responsibility. Only half of the midwives themselves reported giving their notifications to their supervisor. These statistics showed that fewer midwives in this study recognised the role of the supervisor in receiving notifications of intention to practise than in the North West audit where 62 per cent of midwives gave it to their supervisor.

The completion of a notification of intention to practise has received much debate by midwives, supervisors and, probably more vehemently than any other group, the LSA responsible midwifery officers. The UKCC needs a certain amount of information for their database and the LSA officers have other needs. This year, 1999, has produced an excellent form which serves all purposes and has removed a lot of ambiguous terminology. The original purpose of completing the form was to regulate the illiterate midwives at the beginning of the century, but there is still a need today for supervisors to know the details of those on their case-load, as do the LSA responsible midwifery officers to whom they notify their intention to practise.

Practising across trust boundaries

The audit showed that it remained commonplace for midwives to practise across trust boundaries. Midwives worked in this way in all but one trust. Interestingly, in one trust, such midwives had honorary contracts with the trusts in which they might work. The issue of vicarious liability was also a concern for the midwife teachers who were struggling to agree honorary contracts. Similarly, many of the independent midwives faced many barriers, some insurmountable, when endeavouring to get an honorary contract with a trust. This issue may have the knock-on effect of producing barriers for some community midwives wanting to provide continuity of care, as many trust lawyers seek to disclaim vicarious liability for non-trust staff working within a unit.

Arrangements for statutory update and professional development

The audit demonstrated many variables in professional development opportunities. PREP, statutory and clinical supervision all encourage professional development, especially as we move closer to being an all-graduate profession, but the opportunities for professional development appeared to be in decline. Midwives with diplomas or degrees were seen as a threat by some of those without, but some midwives who had tried to embark on courses, found that the funding, which had assisted the colleagues who preceded them, was no longer available. Even giving time for study leave had to be restricted as several midwives wanted to attend college on a certain day and the service could not support the absence of so many midwives on the same day of the week.

It was not unusual to find midwives using their annual leave for study days and the majority funded themselves. A midwife interviewed reported: 'Supervisors of midwives are only able to help in an advisory way. There is no funding for study and to better yourself.' (Midwife site three). Midwives perceived inequity in the way study leave had been allocated:

> We need the motivation to update and have support with professional development, because some people go on all the study days. Supervisors need unbiased views about midwives' need to update, to help them progress and enjoy their work.

The appropriate way forward is for refresher courses, accumulated study days and other study leave to be arranged by the midwife with her supervisor. This was generally found to be the case, but in three units the supervisor continued to make the arrangements and in only one trust was it considered the responsibility of the midwife to arrange her professional updating. Quite remarkably, the trust training officer did not appear to have had influence in statutory update on any of the sites audited. It is of concern, however, that some midwives are not able, or not willing, to take responsibility for their own statutory update. According to many supervisors, it was midwives were unwilling to take this responsibility, hence their charge of 'nannying' as described in the full report (Stapleton, Duerden and Kirkham, 1998). If it is the case that midwives are unwilling to be responsible for their own update, they cannot continue to argue that a midwife is an accountable, autonomous practitioner.

The provision of finance for statutory refresher courses continued to be an issue. Trusts provided either the time or the funding for attendance at accumulated study days, but rarely offered both.

Supervisory reviews

The supervisory review, or annual interview, is considered to be a significant part of the supervisory function (ENB 1996b, ENB 1997) and the supervisory meetings, referred to as 'regular one-to-one sessions' (Butterworth and Faugier, 1992) have a particular emphasis within clinical supervision. All but two of the supervisors in the study carried out such reviews regularly, but the frequency varied, as did the midwives' and supervisors' perceptions of the frequency. There was a tendency for supervisors to report more frequent meetings than did the midwives.

The majority of midwives were able to report meeting with their supervisor and all but one of the midwives working in neonatal units who were interviewed had had a supervisory review within the previous year.

The midwife teachers, however, were not quite so privileged: six had never had a review and only four had met with their supervisor in the preceding year. It appeared that some supervisors felt teachers did not need a supervisory review, or even any supervision. The history of seeing the midwife teachers as somewhat superior, because of their knowledge, may persist into the current day, yet interviews with the teachers demonstrated the complete opposite.

Midwives and supervisors were asked about the duration of supervisory reviews and again perceptions varied, with midwives recalling them as shorter than the supervisors; one midwife believed her last review lasted only five minutes, yet another said hers had taken two and a half hours. None of the supervisors reported either of those extremes, however: the averages were, apart from on one site, fairly close to the anticipated hour (ENB, 1996).

The importance of a supervisory interview taking place in a private environment, free from interruption, was reflected by the vast majority of midwives reporting this to be the case.

The value of the supervisory review was emphasised in some of the commentary, such as this midwife:

> *My supervisor is new and enthusiastic. I was apprehensive about the interview, but soon realised it wasn't as bad as I expected. It is important to review our practice when we are accountable as midwives* (Midwife site one)

and this supervisor:

> *Supervision gives an opportunity for one-to-one: time for encouragement, appreciation and reinforcement.* (Supervisor site one)

There is, as might be expected, still room for improvement as highlighted by another midwife:

> *My last supervisory review had no value. I was told I needed to learn to scrub in order to be able to give total care to a woman.*
> (Independent midwife)

Function of the supervisor

When midwives and supervisors were asked to prioritise the functions of a supervisor in order of importance, it became evident that supervisors were very clear that safeguarding public interest was their most important function, but whether or not the supervisors could actually explain how supervision safeguards the public was not tested. Monitoring safe practice does not guarantee that public interest is safeguarded.

The midwives considered the provision of professional support, guidance and advice for midwives much more important than protecting the public:

Supervision serves a very good purpose, it gives us somebody to approach for advice. (Midwife site one)

No matter how senior you are, it is reassuring to know there is always someone to whom you can refer for reassurance and support. (Midwife site two)

Protecting the public was recognised as important by the midwives, but alongside support:

I think supervision's priority must be the safety of mother and baby first, but close behind that is somebody who will support us. Practice has to be seen to be safe, but it is important to have someone there who can see our side of the coin and knows how we feel. (Midwife site three)

All the midwives were asked how they perceived their supervisors, and the supervisors were asked how they saw themselves as a supervisor, by prioritising from a list of given roles. The results showed that midwives saw their supervisors predominantly as supporters and, indeed, the supervisors saw themselves also in this role. The differing roles, however, were that the supervisors felt they had a strong counselling role, whilst the midwives saw their supervisors more as advisers and guides:

A supervisor is someone who is always there, who listens, understands and never puts you down, and is able to guide you through the problems that you face and come to a satisfactory conclusion. (Midwife site two)

Despite supervision's history of being a disciplinary function, very few saw their supervisors as disciplinarians, although one midwife said:

In the supervisor's eyes we are always guilty. (Midwife site five)

Statutory supervision of midwives as a role model

There remains much confusion about statutory supervision and clinical supervision. When clinical supervision was first introduced, many nursing colleagues were heard to comment that at least the midwives were used to this as they had always had supervision, despite the fact that the clinical model of supervision is very different from what the midwives had received since 1902. When the supervisors, midwives and midwife teachers were all asked if they felt that statutory supervision was a good role model for other professional groups, the majority replied positively. This question did not directly refer to clinical supervision, but it was definitely interpreted that way.

There is much to be commended in clinical supervision in which the supervisor can listen openly, challenge constructively and guide supportively (Deery and Corby, 1996). Hopefully, many supervisors already try to introduce these ideals into their own model of supervision.

On one of the sites, the midwives working in the neonatal unit were offered clinical supervision alongside their statutory supervision and this was well accepted. Another midwife had an idealistic concept of supervision from her husband, a social worker, who had positive experiences of clinical supervision:

> *It would be a dream world for me if I could meet with someone monthly to discuss practice problems.* (Midwife site five)

The need for supervision

There were many negative comments received about supervision in the study, especially during the in-depth interviews by the research midwife; despite this, the overwhelming majority of midwives and midwife teachers believed that midwives need to be supervised. One midwife commented:

> *I mistakenly thought supervision was an authoritarian concept and, having had so much training to make me a responsible practitioner, I didn't need supervision. However, I now see that supervision is a buffer from, and to, the public.* (Midwife site two)

Similarly, when the midwives were asked about the standards of supervision they received, such as identified problems being monitored by their supervisors to ensure that a satisfactory outcome had been reached, receiving the necessary support from their supervisors and the standard of professional information and advice they received, there was always a majority answering in the affirmative, although, as one might expect, many others felt there was room for improvement.

The qualities that midwives valued in a supervisor were prioritised from a given list of ten possible qualities. With hindsight, I would have included confidentiality, but that had not raised its head as an issue in the North West study. Some midwives asked for another quality, that supervisors should have legal knowledge. So much is expected from a supervisor in the nineties, even law degrees it would seem. From the given list, approachability was the most valued quality and clinical experience was also highly valued, along with being in touch and up to date.

Overwhelming need for support

Within this need for supervision was the overwhelming need for support. Help with practice-related problems was highlighted, by the midwives in clinical midwifery practice, as the area in which most support and advocacy was needed. When I carried out the North West audit, the midwives produced long lists detailing the nature of support they would have liked to receive from their supervisors, some realistic but others probably somewhat idealistic considering the amount of time available for supervision within the busy supervisor's workload.

In both studies, midwives articulated how important it was for them simply to know that their supervisor is there for them. Support with professional development was also crucial to many midwives. The list of other support needs was quite amazing. The midwives interviewed identified 101 differing support needs; this was from 170 midwives, compared with the North West study when 170 needs were identified from 357 midwives.

It was possible to group the needs of the individual midwives into: professional development needs; listening and knowing the supervisor is there; help with practice-related problems; help with coping with change (this included team building for some), and conflict; help with client issues such as child protection issues as well as the issues around unreasonable demands from clients; and issues concerning the role of the supervisor. Some midwives were needing support with management issues, which again highlights the difficulties some midwives had in differentiating supervision from management.

Midwives practising outside the NHS

All of the independent midwives were able to detail the issues with which they would value support from a supervisor. As they worked in isolation from the hospital environment, they had their own specific concerns, predominantly their need for recognition in their independent roles. Again, they needed to know the supervisor was there to listen to them, and they wanted her support in dealing with clients whose choice conflicted with their professional judgement as a midwife. Professional development needs were for extended training, such as cannulation, which was not available to midwives outside the hospital service.

Supervision of midwife teachers

When completing the North West study, I learned that many midwife teachers had their own anxieties and would have valued more support from supervisors of midwives. I was, therefore, anxious to ascertain if this group of midwives still experienced the same problems in this later study.

There were considerable differences in the models of supervision available to the midwife teachers interviewed on each site. Site one midwife teachers were based in a university in fairly close proximity to a maternity hospital. They were, therefore, all supervised by the head of midwifery at that unit, even though the majority had their clinical links with other units further afield. Arrangements were not made, however, by that supervisor to meet with the midwife teachers for a supervisory review, or for any other reason. One of the midwife teachers had arranged to meet with her when she had a specific issue to sort out, but there were no formal arrangements for the others.

At two other sites, the midwife teachers were supervised by supervisors in their clinical placement area, which would appear to be the most appropriate type of supervision.

Just eight of the supervisors interviewed said they supervised midwife teachers. In contrast to the North West, these supervisors were not necessarily heads of midwifery and they were valued according to the level of support they offered the teachers and their personal qualities:

The new supervisor has made all the difference. (Midwife teacher site two)

On the whole, I have a good relationship with my supervisor and I feel that a lot of things that crop up are dealt with informally, rather than making a big issue out of them, which is good. (Midwife teacher site four)

Satisfaction was not guaranteed, however, and one supervisor said: 'I have attempted to see my supervisor twice, but have been unsuccessful.' She made the comment that it wasn't needed:

"You're safe." But I feel I am very vulnerable, especially as I work in the clinical area, albeit infrequently, and when I do I am loath to take on difficult cases. (Midwife teacher site three)

This supervisor's comment is extremely worrying when one considers that her predominant role as a supervisor of midwives is to ensure safe practice of midwifery, and here was someone admitting to being concerned about her own clinical practice.

Two of the midwife teachers who were interviewed from the same university did not know their supervisor. The issues that some of the teachers had wanted to raise with their supervisor included delivering a friend's baby, discussion prior to clinical placement, career advice and to discuss the practice of another midwife.

Despite the fact that we learned it was rather unusual, nowadays, for supervisors to carry out planned observation of practice, one of the midwife teachers had received planned observation from a supervisor, during her practice placement two years earlier, for a period of four hours.

The midwife teachers inevitably had their own, if differing, support needs from their supervisor. For the majority, as in the North West, these needs revolved around their concerns about their eligibility to practise as a midwife. Eleven of the midwife teachers interviewed considered themselves practising midwives, but four did not. Even though four teachers felt they were not practising midwives, all but one felt they should sign notification of intention to practise.

The teachers described how they kept updated with clinical practice whilst working in academic institutions. This varied from reading journals and attending study days, to receiving feedback from students and colleagues. Some undertook annual clinical placement whilst others tried to fit in practice days. The lecturer practitioners were best placed with their appointments providing 50 per cent practice.

As with the other groups of midwives, the midwife teachers expressed support needs which again reflected the desire to know that the supervisor is there to listen. They, too, had issues regarding professional practice, especially enlisting support with their practitioner role, to enable them to get back into practice. There was also the need to talk to supervisors about student issues. Both the teachers and the students were having to come to terms with the long distances between the academic institutions and the practice placements. Many of the issues are expressed by this midwife teacher:

> *Since NHS trusts, continuous assessment programmes, and latterly the university, the workload and responsibilities have mitigated against clinical link work. The distance of link areas also precludes ad hoc visits, therefore spare time can not be used in the same way it used to be when on a hospital site. It weakens links between education and practice and subsequently my credibility as a midwife teacher.* (Midwife teacher site one)

At the time of the audit, the problem of vicarious liability for midwife teachers working in trust premises was not resolved. This caused much concern for many and is described here by a midwife teacher from site four:

> *Our honorary contracts are not yet drawn up, and we are expected to be in the clinical area, but we are not covered by insurance to do anything.*

Supervision of midwives working in neonatal units

It had been clear during the former study that these midwives had their own particular needs from supervision which were not being met. Eleven midwives working in neonatal units on three sites were interviewed: all knew their supervisor and the majority had met with their supervisor in the previous year, most within the last six months. The exceptions were the two who had not met with their supervisor in the past two years. Once again, the biggest concern for this group of midwives was their eligibility to practise as midwives, as described by a midwife from site four:

> *As a midwife working in the neonatal unit, I am concerned about losing my title of midwife. I worked long and hard to get it. I would like the support of my supervisor to ensure I retain my role as a midwife.*

Five of the midwives interviewed rotated out into the maternity unit to update in midwifery practice and enable them to notify their intention to practise as a midwife. For the remaining midwives, there were very few opportunities to achieve this practice experience, although two were able to help on the labour ward or in other areas of the maternity unit when the neonatal unit was quiet, three midwives were on the midwifery bank, and one participated in parent education.

At the present time, 12 weeks of midwifery practice are required in each five year period. From April 2000, every midwife will have to have practised midwifery for 100 days in the preceding five year period (ENB, 1996a; UKCC, 1996) to avoid undertaking a return to midwifery practice course.

As neonatal units have become part of paediatric rather than obstetric, directorates,midwives are not supported by the managers in rotating into the maternity unit because of staffing issues. This has meant that such midwives have to determine whether they want to return to substantive posts in the maternity department or remain neonatal nurses. All the midwives interviewed defended their eligibility to practise by the advice they gave to mothers and babies and, for some, this was hands-on care as they looked after mothers who were 'rooming-in' on the neonatal unit.

The support needs from supervisors for this group of midwives were grouped into professional development needs, including career guidance and support with rotation, and listening. Some of the support they needed fell under the management umbrella, which was of concern if the role of the supervisor was inadequately recognised.

Conclusion

Results from this audit proved to be little different from that in the North West, with many recurring themes. There appeared to be a greater desire for midwives to seek out their supervisors for advice and many midwives spoke of supervision having an increased profile in recent years. A strong feature of this study was the need for support from supervisors in the changing world of the NHS, with a longing to be heard and to have someone to off-load to as the overwhelming support need. This need for support was probably the reason that the vast majority of midwives believed there was a need for supervision.

The specific needs of midwives, teachers and midwives working in neonatal units were investigated and identified, as were those of independent midwives, and there is much work to be done in each of these areas.

It was difficult to identify specific models of supervision within each trust, but supervisory activities complied with guidelines in most, although there were inconsistencies.

The supervisor:midwife ratio is reducing as supervisor appointments increase. Midwives were able to contact a supervisor 24 hours a day. The days of midwives not knowing if they had a supervisor appear to be long gone; without exception the midwives who could not identify their supervisor were newly appointed or newly qualified.

The development of the LSA responsible midwifery officer role has provided much more contact for supervisors.

The demands for support from midwives appear so great that there must be concern that some supervisors may not be able to provide that support, although the majority of midwives felt they received the support they needed from their supervisor. Approachability was prioritised as the quality most valued in a supervisor; to seek such support this quality is vital. It can be of no surprise that the midwives believed that giving professional support was the most important function of a supervisor, whilst safeguarding the public was considered the most important function by the supervisors.

The old-fashioned image of supervisors appears to have gone as they were rarely perceived as disciplinarians, monitors, preceptors or friends. The majority of midwives saw their supervisors as supporters, advisers, guides and counsellors. Midwives wanted to be involved in the selection of supervisors in their trust, presumably hoping they will be able to select midwives with the qualities needed to be a supportive supervisor in the pressured world of midwifery.

References

Butterworth, C.A., Faugier, J. (1992). *Clinical Supervision and Mentorship in Nursing*. London: Chapman and Hall.
Department of Health (1995). Executive Letter EL(95) 77 NHSE.
Department of Health (1993). *Changing Childbirth*. London: HMSO.

Deery, R., Corby, D. (1996). A case for Clinical Supervision in Midwifery. In: Kirkham, M.J. (ed.) *Supervision of Midwives*. Hale: Books for Midwives Press

Duerden, J. (1995). *Audit of Supervision of Midwives in the North West Regional Health Authority*. Salford Royal Hospitals NHS Trust DMI.

Duerden, J. (1997). 'Supervisors' and midwives' morale in the NHS.' *Modern Midwife* Vol. 7, No. 5, pp. 15-19.

ENB (1996a). *Return to Practice Guidelines for Programmes: Leading to the Renewal of Registration and Re-entry to Registered Practice*. London: ENB.

ENB (1996b). *Supervision of Midwives: The English National Board's Advice and Guidance to Local Supervising Authorities and Supervisors of Midwives*. London: ENB.

ENB (1997). Preparation of Supervision of Midwives: An open learning programme. London: ENB.

Stapleton, H., Duerden J., Kirkham M. (1998). *Evaluation of the Impact of the Supervision of Midwives on Professional Practice and the Quality of Midwifery Care*. London: ENB.

Thomas, M., Mayes, G. (1996). The ENB perspective: preparation of supervisors of midwives for their role. In: Kirkham M.J. (ed.) *Supervision of Midwives*. Hale: Books for Midwives Press.

UKCC (1996). Registrar's Letter 7/1996.

Helen Stapleton • Mavis Kirkham

Supervision of Midwives
England 1996-7

RESEARCH AND AUDIT

Method

The qualitative part of the study took an ethnographic approach and 168 in-depth interviews were conducted with midwives and supervisors drawn from all grades and practice settings on six sites. Midwives were asked to reflect upon their practice and supervision and, when assured of the confidentiality of the interview and the anonymity of the data, they did so with considerable insight. Focus groups were also held with service users and student midwives on the study sites and with supervisors elsewhere.

The style of the study appeared best suited to a grounded theory approach in its analysis (Glaser and Strauss, 1967). Such an approach allows for the emergence and continual evolution of theoretical frameworks in synchrony with the actual research. The interview transcripts were selectively coded and the emerging categories were constantly explored in the ongoing interviews and analysis. Whilst some categories collapsed or merged, others appeared; this process went on until no further 'movement' of categories was detected. Thus, the researchers felt confident that the categories had reached the point of 'saturation' (Strauss and Corbin, 1990).

Findings

This qualitative analysis is primarily concerned with evaluating the influence of supervision on midwifery practice and analysing those elements of supervision which contributed significantly to the quality of care delivered to mothers and babies. Since the influence of supervision on care is mediated through its influence upon the midwives who deliver that care, it was examined through the views of the midwives interviewed. Where very small, or very large, numbers of midwives expressed an opinion about supervision, this is stated in the text. Where this is not stated, the issue was raised by a considerable number of midwives on all sites, unless a specific statement is made with regard to site.

Approaches to supervision

As well as the different, and constantly evolving, philosophies of supervision, other factors appeared to profoundly influence, and direct, supervision on each of the sites studied. These factors were:

- the culture of midwifery

- midwives' past experience of, and learned reactions to, supervision

- the way in which supervision was perceived by supervisees and interpreted by supervisors

- the dilemmas inherent within supervision

- the organisational power structures within which supervision operated.

The factors listed above were constantly manifest in the data. They overlap considerably in the issues examined and the structure of this chapter aims to bring out that complexity.

In illustrating themes in this analysis, attention is focused on particular sites where local conditions brought an issue to the fore. This is done in order to add the depth of a case study approach to the analysis and to gain full benefit from the use of grounded theory. Nevertheless, issues described here were found on all sites unless stated otherwise. To ensure confidentiality, some quotations are not attributed by site.

Supervision as a professional characteristic of midwifery

Many midwives saw supervision as a factor differentiating midwifery from other professions and, as such, it seemed an important feature in maintaining a separate professional identity.

> *I just think it's something midwives should cling onto like mad because it's something that distinguishes us from the nursing profession.* (Newly qualified midwife site four)

> *We are privileged to have supervision... there is nothing like it in nursing or medicine... doctors should have it as well... I think it makes our practice much more respected because we can be seen to be really looking at how to improve ourselves... supervisors can get to the root of the problems.* (G grade community midwife site one)

These comments should not be read as uniformly positive statements about supervision per se, rather as the consistency of opinion related to how midwives perceived supervision with specific regard to the maintenance and exclusivity of professional status.

The culture of midwifery in the NHS

Service, sacrifice and lack of support

A clear picture of the culture of midwifery in the NHS emerged from the midwives' detailed descriptions of the context of their practice (for a more detailed analysis of this culture see Stapleton, Duerden and Kirkham 1998, and Kirkham 1999). This is a female culture of caring expressed through service and sacrifice. This caring takes place within institutions with very different, culturally coded, values which do not acknowledge the importance of such caring work. Therefore, whilst midwives gave care, their role as professional carer discounted their need for personal and professional support. In recent years, changes in the maternity services have encouraged women to expect appropriate care and support as a right. Midwives, however, did not perceive themselves as having parallel rights. In some cases this deficit was reinforced by powerful role models:

> *Any model of women centred care doesn't help midwives to think about their own needs because in that culture midwives aren't seen as women – they're seen as the 'lead professional'... It's important to think about the women but we're important too... And you've got to get that balance right because if you get midwives stressed out and burnt out then it affects the care for these women. That's one criticism I would make of B [supervisor] – she is so nice and enthusiastic about everything that she sometimes puts us in a difficult position where we're expected to be as self sacrificing as she is... so when we're short staffed and someone comes in labour, B just tells us to carry on because she doesn't want to bother anybody else to call them in... And what can you say when she's prepared to do it?* (F grade site four)

As well as a lack of role models of support, midwives experienced a lack of mutual support:

> *We don't support each other... we don't ever stand up for each other.* (G grade site four)

Guilt and blame

Such a culture, with deeply internalised values of service and self-sacrifice, produced considerable guilt and blame. Self-blame was widespread and, whilst this may be a female characteristic in the wider culture surrounding midwifery, it had an undermining effect upon midwives:

> ... *no matter how much I go through it, I know nobody can be blamed, but at the back of your mind you think it must have been your fault... it must have been something you did or something you didn't do.* (F grade site one)

It is noteworthy that many respondents, when invited to reflect on the need for support and on ways of looking after themselves, used the word 'selfish'. Thus, the word chosen by midwives seeking to address their own needs, was itself an indictment in the caring, self-sacrificing, client-centred culture.

> *So I think we really need to be thinking about ourselves and be selfish at times really. But that really goes against the grain in midwifery.* (F grade site four)

A few midwives, in the privacy of the research interview, spoke of private resolutions to protect their own health. Such resolutions were not voiced easily, nor without an accompanying sense of guilt; they were, therefore, unlikely to be implemented because of the strong resistance within the prevailing culture.

Midwives interviewed made constant allusions to blame. Often this blame was directed inwardly at themselves, sometimes towards a midwife perceived as deviant within that culture and sometimes towards managers, supervisors or clients. Where such blame was acted out on colleagues, it fits the definition of horizontal violence (Fanon, 1963).

Horizontal violence is not just a description of inter-group conflict or various forms of 'bullying'; it embodies an understanding of how oppressed groups direct their frustrations and dissatisfactions towards each other as a response to a system that has excluded them from power (Leap, 1997).

Learned helplessness and muting

In such a context, many midwives voiced a resigned acceptance of their lot and a low sense of their own worth. The general tone of their comments was of an overwhelming sense of helplessness and of low expectations.

Midwives described a professional setting within which their voices were muted or silenced. Experience of a culture of powerlessness left midwives ill-equipped to empower their clients, because they lacked the confidence or sense of their own power that is needed before power can be shared.

Within the culture of midwifery, it was difficult, but not impossible, for midwives to bring about change. This was often achieved, however, in complex and devious ways which appeared not to challenge the existing culture. This 'doing good by stealth' (independent midwife) could bring about change in particular circumstances but, as it was concealed, it did not lead to concerted action or major change. Only on rare occasions did midwives and supervisors attempt to challenge this culture in more open ways.

The market, management and the culture of midwifery

In recent years, the pressures of market forces in the NHS have reinforced the more oppressive aspects of the culture of midwifery. Midwives described general management as oppressive on site three and in one unit within site four.

> There is a real fear that if we don't provide good care, and look after them [clients] really well, they won't come back and that the unit will close... but I think we go a bit overboard really. (F grade site four)

On site three, which served as a case study of aggressive, modern management, these pressures were so great as to dwarf the pressures from the culture of midwifery. Whilst general management has an impact on all NHS employees, the interface with supervision was particularly significant on this site.

> ... the environment for midwives is becoming more and more stressful and it seems unfair to expect them to have to cope, but the ones who don't, just get dealt with by management because when you are stressed and not handling it well, it often shows in behaviour... It's a big problem in the health services – not just in midwifery – and I don't know how we deal with it... it seems that in some places supervision is not able to protect midwives very much from management. (HoM site three)

The possibility of change

The features of the culture of midwifery outlined above were described repeatedly. That is not to imply that change was seen as impossible, but it did suggest that many factors worked against it being viewed positively by many respondents. Nonetheless, examples of successful change were identified which were recognised as inspiring by the respondents involved. The supervision philosophy in practice on site two was seen as a model of successful innovation in this respect. It was felt to be helpful in facilitating midwives to learn the skills of challenging, of evidence-based argument, and of professional empowerment within the safe setting of supervision. There were other supervisors on sites one and five who were similarly praised by their supervisees for sharing a philosophy of supervision which was experienced as empowering. These supervisors had considerable influence in negotiating change and in ensuring that this was achieved with the minimum of disruption for the midwives they supervised.

Midwives and supervision

Midwives' knowledge of supervision

The majority of midwives interviewed demonstrated a lack of knowledge about supervision. This included its official purpose and function and the framework within which it operates. The nomination, selection and deselection of supervisors, together with the evaluation and monitoring of their role, were also areas about which the majority of respondents knew very little. These areas are explored in the full report (Stapleton, Duerden and Kirkham, 1998).

The midwives who were knowledgeable about supervision included those practising outside the NHS, midwives who had gained knowledge through being involved in an incident investigated by a supervisor or a manager, and those supervisors who had completed the ENB distance learning programme. There was no evidence that the knowledge of supervision held by senior students and newly qualified midwives was any greater than that of midwives who qualified some years ago.

This lack of knowledge is perhaps not surprising. Supervision may have been a statutory obligation for almost 100 years, but it is only in very recent years that it has had any real meaning for the majority of practising midwives.

Midwives' views on the function and purpose of supervision

Despite their lack of knowledge and understanding of the subject, when given the opportunity to consider the function and purpose of supervision, midwives were generally eloquent in discussing this from the basis of their professional experience.

Initially, many volunteered that the purpose of supervision was 'to protect the public' but, upon further reflection, they often stated that this was now achieved by other means. The need for the supervisor to protect the midwife was raised on every site. Sometimes this was seen as protection in the face of increasing levels of complaints and litigation:

> ... *because as midwives we are more out on a limb legally. We do need that support.* (Newly qualified midwife site five)

Often this plea for support was combined with a plea for protection, both within the midwifery culture and within the wider organisational culture. The latter was widely regarded by respondents from all grades as swift to blame and to punish.

Many midwives spoke about their efforts to implement woman centred care, often in situations where midwifery management failed to recognise that midwives needed to be supported and facilitated if they were to provide a good standard of care to clients. Midwives' need for advocacy, for someone with 'clout' who would support them in the wider management arena, was also raised by respondents on all sites.

Respondents' differing views on the purpose, or function, of supervision reflected what they understood to be their professional needs. These were often tempered by their earlier experiences of supervision and it was from these relationships that subsequent expectations were developed about what was, and what was not, possible within supervision.

> Interviewer: *What do you gain from your yearly review with your supervisor?*
>
> *Not a lot. I've also had a couple of clinical sessions where I've been watched doing a basic skill like talking to a woman in labour... I didn't find it helpful – just embarrassing and I'm sure the supervisor didn't get anything out of it either! I think that kind of thing is just irrelevant.* (E grade site five)

The most important thing I've got out of it [supervision] *is that it's quite inspirational when people appear interested in you. It may give you the extra encouragement that you might need... so that spurs me on to think about other things... I feel quite motivated to do my study days and some courses... I feel very motivated to keep updated in the clinical area.* (F grade site five)

Interviewer: *What purpose does supervision serve for you?*

Well basically you really need somebody to make you realise what you really want to do; like where you're going and the best way to go about getting there... you really need someone to help you to get to where you want to go. (E grade site five)

Positive experiences of supervision enabled midwives to have positive, and appropriately high, expectations of their supervisor. Such experiences, especially if held by a number of midwives, also served to raise the general profile of supervision within the unit and this was particularly noticeable on sites two and five. Negative experience of supervision, however, marked midwives deeply and also curbed future expectations.

The power imbalance within the supervisory relationship was felt by some respondents to undermine the supportive function of supervision:

Interviewer: *So you wouldn't think of a supervisor as being your counsellor or guide... as someone you could turn to for support?*

No... absolutely not... never. No, not at all... Those words are so naive... if anything serious like that was happening in my professional life supervisors would be the last people I would speak to... Family and friends are for that... I agree that's what it's meant to be but no, I'd never use supervisors for that. (F grade site five)

Many midwives saw supervision as still primarily concerned with monitoring practice. The exceptions were midwives on site two and those midwives supervised directly by the HoM on site five who experienced supervision as aiding their professional development.

A large number of respondents appeared to derive considerable comfort from the monitoring and policing aspects of supervision. This seemed to give midwives a feeling of safety and protection, particularly from low standards of practice on the part of colleagues. This aspect of supervision also afforded them a sense of security against the threat of litigation. It appeared that it was only when supervisors had successfully contradicted midwives' negative perceptions that any real change was possible with regard to their current understanding of either the function, or purpose, of supervision. This was not easy as the resistance put up by midwives often required that the supervisor put considerable effort into challenging their prejudices and stereotypes.

Respondents from all grades expected considerable amounts of 'nannying' from supervisors, particularly concerning requirements for their refresher courses and in making arrangements for their ongoing professional development. It could be argued, however, that these are obligations which a member of any other profession would be expected to fulfil themselves.

Some midwives and supervisors expressed the opinion that these expectations were more widely held because of the recent increase in numbers of available supervisors. Not all supervisors accepted these expectations as reasonable, however:

> We have to not encourage them into feeling that we can do everything for them. (G grade supervisor site five)

Some supervisors, who were trying hard to implement changes within supervision, occasionally reported feeling threatened by midwives when they refused to accommodate their (unrealistic) expectations. In working toward reducing unnecessary dependency, supervisors appreciated that the very elements which encouraged it were well embedded into the role. This may have made it difficult for supervisors to challenge even those situations where overt dependency appeared to be causing problems in the supervisory relationship.

The enabling aspects of supervision are emphasised over the inspectoral role in recent literature (ENB, 1997). It takes a long time, however, for change to permeate through the layers of any organisation and as the literature describing many of the changes to supervision has generally been available only to senior members of the midwifery profession, it may take even longer for midwives to respond.

The attributes and skills considered important in a supervisor

Supervisors and supervisees were asked to describe what they considered to be the important characteristics of a good supervisor. Sometimes these were constructed directly from their experience and from what they thought to be practicable, but on many occasions the descriptions represented idealised notions.

A large proportion of the midwives interviewed felt that supervisors should have recent clinical experience, 'otherwise I wouldn't trust them' (E grade site five). It was also felt to be very important that a supervisor was approachable. Approachability was a factor which was often linked with clinical skills because increasing numbers of clinically based supervisors were working alongside their supervisees:

> *The qualities which are important to me in a supervisor are confidentiality, approachability, motivation and a real ability to encompass the individual needs of staff... an ability to put herself in my shoes and see it the way I do.* (G grade lecturer-practitioner site five)

In addition to the widely cited attribute of 'approachability', rather more elusive 'interpersonal skills' were reiterated by a number of respondents as being of considerable importance in a supervisor. These skills included an ability to balance the complex, and infinitely variable, pressures upon her, as well as empowering and acting as an advocate for the midwives she supervised. Skills in advocacy, change agency, adjudication and conflict resolution were also seen as important for effective supervision. This was a noticeable feature of site five where one supervisor was regarded as exemplary in taking an active stance by encouraging midwives initially to draw on their own resources in order to resolve problems and conflict:

> *Supervisors as women have to be strong and they have to know who they are defending and why. They have to feel they are capable of supporting other women... but they also have to know they have backing when they are addressing difficult issues. Over the years women have been disempowered and they need midwives a lot more but midwives also have been disempowered so I suppose that is where supervisors could come in – to empower the midwives. It is hectic down there on CDS... it's quite dangerous at times so you start to practise defensively instead of in a caring and compassionate way... supervisors have to really love and care about the midwives.* (G grade site five)

> *I'd say my supervisor is a good communicator and a good listener... she triggers off the right sort of thoughts.* (E grade site five)

The expectations midwives had of supervisors revealed many assumptions made about the innate talents, or acquired skills, of supervisors. There are parallels between the skills valued in supervision and those which maternity service users raised as important with regard to the skills and attributes of the midwives caring for them. Highly developed and flexible skills in empathy and support were clearly seen by service users as important in clinical midwifery and by midwives as important in supervision.

Confidentiality and confidence

Confidentiality was of key importance to supervisees. The interview data showed that supervisees who had experienced breaches of confidentiality no longer trusted supervisors with any information considered to be of value. Changing supervisors was not usually seen as a solution because, in such cases, it appeared that all supervisors everywhere were collectively mistrusted by the respondent concerned.

> *... we've all got supervisors in units – and unfortunately they are often in quite senior positions – who just aren't capable of keeping confidences. So you can hardly blame the midwives for not accessing supervision can you?... but it's the midwives who do get the blame for not being more proactive about accessing supervision because we don't have effective systems for monitoring the behaviour of supervisors... we monitor a bit of what they do now but not how they do it.* (Trainee supervisor site one)

Breaches in confidentiality were universally regarded by midwives as being the point at which trust broke down and this effectively reduced further contact between both parties to a minimum.

Midwives had to be able to trust the supervisor in order to feel safe to reveal concerns to her. Some supervisors were felt to be intimidating, and this was another factor which made confidence impossible. In order to trust the supervisor, the midwife had to feel safe within the supervisory relationship. This was one of the reasons why many midwives felt such ambivalence about being supervised by their manager and why supervisors who did not hold a management position were generally seen as more trustworthy.

The link between trust, self-confidence and confidentiality was complex, as was highlighted after the suspension of a senior midwife on site one. This action was experienced by many respondents as a major rupturing of the social order, with midwives of all grades left feeling threatened and vulnerable. Impeccable standards of confidentiality were certainly maintained, but this led other midwives to feel anxious and threatened.

> *... it's really knocked us badly. So everyone at the moment is feeling a bit low and wary. The trouble is that nobody really knows the full story behind it. I think actually that may be the problem. Perhaps if the full story came out, it may reassure people more. At the moment we have only one side of the story – the midwife's side. If we could get it from the supervision side, a lot of the anxieties and mistrusts might disappear.* (G grade site one)

> *It's just really who you can trust and will it happen to me? But I think it's also one of those areas that is very difficult because of the confidentiality thing. They are trying to arrange for us to have some debriefing sessions... I think that would be good as I do feel that is an important part of the supervisor's role because if you get this mistrust going round, it affects morale, and that affects the care we give to women.* (F grade site one)

The suspension of a colleague was perceived as a threat akin to bereavement; self-blame and guilt appeared to be common reactions and many respondents were aware that these feelings affected their practice. The professional confidence of midwives on site one could therefore be said to be undermined by these reactions. Thus, at least within the culture of midwifery on this site, both the observance and the breach of confidentiality were experienced as undermining for midwives.

For supervisors too, confidentiality was a difficult issue. The majority of supervisees perceived the individual supervisor as the ultimate keeper of all that was disclosed. Supervisors, for their part, did not seem to question this, nor did they see it as inappropriate in any way, despite a number of them commenting on the personal cost of this 'unexpected burden of responsibility'.

Clearly the issues of confidentiality, and its impact upon midwives' confidence, are complex and subtle. There are many ways in which the supervisor's actions can make the midwife vulnerable and dealing with, or pre-empting, that experience of vulnerability, requires great skill. The degree to which respondents were willing to make themselves vulnerable through disclosure about issues which concerned them was largely determined by their estimate of the receptiveness of the supervisor. In addition to this, her ability to contain what was revealed, both in terms of knowledge of the event and of the associated emotions, was also mentioned as important. Where this was achieved, whether directly as a result of the skills of the individual supervisor, or by directing the supervisee to a more appropriate person, it was reported to positively affect the supervisee's relationships with her clients. The responsibilities upon the supervisor are clearly great, but the opportunities for learning interpersonal skills within her own supervision are limited.

Supervision for less 'visible' midwives

With the many pressures on supervisors' time, it is easy to understand why midwives in minority groups were often not supervised, or were supervised in a way which did not meet their particular needs. There is cause for professional concern that midwives working in isolated positions, who are particularly likely to need support, are those least likely to receive supervision.

> *The groups of midwives I feel particularly concerned about are those working as agency midwives, the independent midwives, those working on the bank and the practice nurses... all those midwives who are external to the establishment and who are not being looked after at all... who are just invisible as far as supervision is concerned.* (LSA officer)

Most agency midwives interviewed received no formal supervision, though they felt themselves to be in a stressful and vulnerable position.

Midwifery lecturers were another group frequently excluded from supervisory arrangements. Many lecturers, especially those with little recent clinical experience, expressed anxieties about their clinical competence, particularly as a number of them had recently been pressured to take a higher profile in the clinical area, but without any supervisory support. This situation was echoed by many other midwives in specialist posts such as researchers, genetic counsellors, infant feeding advisers and ultrasonographers, as many felt that their needs were not currently being addressed by supervision.

A small number of respondents were employed in a private hospital and were supervised from a local NHS provider unit. The issues they raised were similar to other midwives working outside of the mainstream. They also valued supervisor support relevant to their needs, rather than the needs of the NHS.

The self-employed midwives interviewed described, in some detail, the various attempts they had made to resolve the issue of finding appropriate supervision. The interviews with these midwives echoed many of the comments of their NHS colleagues but they also produced sharp contrasts in their descriptions of alternative models of the supervisory relationship. The wide geographical area in which independent midwives practised afforded them a more global perspective with regard to the differences between supervisors.

These respondents appeared particularly vulnerable with respect to the absence of any formal mechanism for appealing against decisions taken by supervisors. They also felt vulnerable when supervisors appeared uninformed about, and uninterested in, their practice. Sometimes this was felt to result from the supervisor confusing her responsibilities and attempting to manage, rather than supervise, these midwives.

Some supervisors did endeavour to support independent midwives, but found this difficult because of the power relationships with, and loyalties towards, their employing agency. They therefore resorted to 'doing good by stealth', usually with very limited results.

Unlike their NHS colleagues, midwives practising outside the NHS rarely saw supervisors as a primary source of support. They consciously drew support from many sources including their immediate colleagues, their clients and from other health professionals. It is significant that these relationships were also used to monitor their practice through direct feedback from one another, but within a safe environment. They were clearly operating in a very different culture from that of midwifery in the NHS.

The different attitude these non-NHS midwives displayed towards supervision was striking, but it was not possible to discern whether, or how much, this difference resulted from the nurturing they received from their strong support systems. Whatever the reasons, this group of midwives did hold quite different expectations of the supervisory function and appeared more pragmatic with regard to the limitations of the supervisor's role.

Reformulating negative experiences

A number of respondents described themselves as being marked in some way by previous negative encounters with supervision. These memories appeared to make it difficult for midwives to trust that a positive experience could be possible. The turning point for supervisees, with regard to the moderating of distorted or negative perceptions of supervision, appeared to be through direct contact with an individual supervisor who clearly valued them.

Respondents on sites where supervisors had put on workshops, seminars and roadshows on the subject of supervision, did comment that these events had been helpful in 'raising awareness levels'. For those midwives who had been disciplined however, educational forums such as these appeared to increase their knowledge about supervision, but also served to reinforce their memories of earlier, painful experiences. Hence the (negative) perceptions of supervision for these respondents remained relatively unchanged. It was primarily through direct contact with a supervisor who was able to demonstrate qualities such as the ability to hold confidences and to respect and affirm the midwife in her work, that any resolution of these earlier experiences was seen to be possible.

There appeared to be direct parallels between midwives and their clients in terms of reformulating previous negative experiences. In each situation similar professional skills and attitudes appeared to be needed to allow 'old ways of knowing' (Belenky et al, 1986) to be challenged. On the occasions when respondents felt safe to voice accounts of previous difficult experiences, an opportunity was created whereby the past could be reinterpreted, and the future anticipated more hopefully. Supervision has the potential to create a safe environment wherein misconceptions and beliefs are challenged; it could also be the field which supports midwives and, by extension, mothers in their care, in the right to hold opinions which contradict the 'absolutist dictates of the authorities', in favour of their own subjective experiences (Belenky et al, 1986). If this challenge could be sustained, it might go some way towards transforming this present culture of punishment and blame.

Choice of supervisor

The majority of midwives interviewed wanted to choose their supervisor although very few currently had that choice. Whilst midwives could change supervisors, few did, even when they admitted to difficulties in the relationship. The main reasons given for this were concerns about upsetting the supervisor's feelings; being seen as 'difficult' and having to suffer the associated consequences; and the homogeneity of the philosophies and approaches on offer within the unit or geographical isolation with rural units being supervised by a single supervisor. Only independent midwives appeared relatively untroubled about changing to a different supervisor.

Some midwives were concerned, however, that they did not have sufficient information to make a choice of supervisor:

> We should be able to choose our supervisor; you have to be able to relate to them and rely on and trust them and you can't do that with someone you know nothing about. (E grade site four)

The Practice of Supervision

Old and new styles of supervision: dilemmas and role models

The majority of midwives interviewed, and certainly all the hospital midwives, had only been aware of the function of supervision in recent years. Several supervisors admitted that they had become more attentive to supervision only during their training to become supervisors.

The current training of supervisors was generally seen as a great improvement. However, few of the supervisors interviewed had had the experience of being well supervised before they became supervisors, and very few of them had any role model who might guide them through the period of transition to becoming supervisors.

In situations where change is a pivotal feature, role modelling is of key importance. Inevitably, at the inception of a training programme which is attempting to prepare supervisors for a new, and more enabling, style of supervision, those with the necessary skills to guide the trainees through this transition are in short supply. The mentors to the current generation of trainee, and newly qualified, supervisors were educated to deliver the old model of supervision. It will, therefore, take some time before there are sufficient numbers of supervisors trained in the new style to acquire the confidence and the power to make any impact. All of these factors appeared to have acted as a brake upon effecting measurable change within supervision. The LSA officers were particularly vocal on this issue.

> *When I look at all the newly qualified supervisors, all I see is that they might have been very well prepared for their role but all they are actually doing on the ground is replicating the role as it has been practised in their unit or the neighbouring unit... I've listened to the new supervisors around here and I know they've got ideas as to how they'd like to supervise but I'm not seeing those ideas being acted on. So I'm not seeing a lot in the way of what you might call innovative styles... I'm not sure whether it's to do with the hierarchy or whether it's about lack of good role models... but whatever the reason I find it very depressing.* (LSA officer)

Superimposed upon these dilemmas in the preparation of supervisors was the fact that a number of the supervisors interviewed were not themselves currently receiving supervision and others had only recent, and limited, experience of being supervised. Thus, at a time when the expectations of supervision are rising, many supervisors have very limited skills and little experience upon which they can draw. Despite this deficit, some newly qualified supervisors did try to change the local practice of supervision, but often felt very isolated in these endeavours.

> *One of the most difficult things has been working in a unit where I am the only one to have done the new course and the other supervisors don't seem to be that interested in doing things differently. It's been really hard not having a like-minded person to refer to.* (G grade supervisor)

Tensions between the old and new styles of supervision appeared to be an issue for supervisors in most of the units researched. The manifestation of this tension was most commonly expressed as the newly qualified, or trainee, supervisor experiencing some degree of resistance from those who had been in post for some years.

Some of the older generation of supervisors appeared threatened by this new wave of well-trained, and knowledgeable, supervisors. This threat has, of course, been echoed in clinical practice with the advent of graduate midwives.

Some midwives also reported difficulties in accepting supervision from a former colleague and/or peer, especially if this midwife was younger, or had less midwifery experience. Midwives wanted supervisors to be accessible and approachable, yet these attributes were not universally appreciated, perhaps because they contradicted some of the more invisible aspects of the supervisor's role. A degree of separation from colleagues was thought, by many respondents, to be necessary in order to fulfil some of the less attractive aspects of the role. Some respondents drew attention to the personal barriers they encountered when required to invest a clinical colleague, and a former peer, with the very authority which they also saw as an essential quality in a supervisor.

There was a distinct picture of supervisors as not being 'one of us', and having different priorities from those of clinical midwives. Even where efforts were made to ensure that a newly qualified supervisor was not put in an invidious position, resentment was still occasionally expressed. The transition from midwife to supervisor was not always an easy one.

Some supervisors newly in post were acutely aware of the difficulties involved in taking on this role within a highly conservative, professional, culture:

> *I am really aware of the need to maintain the momentum of the changes going on in supervision at the moment... I hope it won't be knocked out of us. There is a lot of keen blood around and we need to be really careful that the older traditional supervisors don't monopolise supervision... because of our roots and background the sense of hierarchy and tradition is very strong in midwifery and that makes it hard to change established ways of doing things.* (Newly qualified supervisor)

Thus, the changes in supervision which were widely seen as empowering for supervisees appeared to reinforce feelings of isolation, loneliness and vulnerability in newly qualified supervisors. The difficulties in adapting to this new supervisory role extended to LSA level.

Intimidation

Some midwives found their experience of supervision intimidating and, whilst very few used the word 'bullying' of supervision, research shows the potential for the abuse of power in midwifery (RCM, 1996).

Accusations can only be reported as the perceptions of those concerned; however, they also suggest that the autonomy bestowed upon supervisors cannot always be regarded as necessarily benign. A supervisor of midwives commands an authority to make decisions with which her supervisees may disagree, but with which they will probably comply, out of deference to her more powerful position.

> ... *there's no way as a midwife you can contradict what a supervisor says.* (F grade)

None of the respondents who stated they felt intimidated by a supervisor reported having confronted her about this. Nor were there formal, and effective, mechanisms for local appeal against supervisory decisions.

Some midwives described how colleagues colluded with the pressure put upon an individual by the supervisor concerned:

> ... *she's a real bully... so the other midwives often end up supporting her not because they agree with her but because they are afraid of her and as it's a very small unit, she has quite a lot of control.* (F grade)

In these situations midwives occasionally gave the impression that there was collusion higher in the managerial and supervision structures:

> *So eventually I couldn't take it any longer and spoke to the HoM at the DGH about it and she was very supportive in helping me change supervisor but she didn't tackle the problem which I'm very disappointed about...* [another midwife] *appealed to the supervisors at the DGH but they wouldn't get involved – kept on about supervisors being autonomous – so eventually the midwife left the unit.* (F grade)

What is seen as collusion with bullying by a supervisee can thus be seen as fostering supervisory autonomy by those in a management position.

Some supervisors were aware of their own power in these situations:

> *You've got so much power over them when you're in this role so you need to be really careful when you appoint somebody especially because you are in post for so long.* (H grade supervisor)

There were also variations in the willingness to be explicit:

Bullying is a strong word. It's more the impression that there are brick walls and unreceptive minds and that some managers and supervisors feel threatened if people question what they are doing or even if they express a different opinion. (LSA officer)

Local factors suggest that midwives' feelings of intimidation may have resulted from supervisors feeling threatened by change; from having supervisees whose views opposed their own; or because the supervisor had neither the ability, nor the skills, to deal effectively with conflict or stress.

Differing expectations and philosophies between supervisors and supervisees could be perceived as oppressive in both directions. The positional power invested in the supervisor's role allowed the supervisor to tell the supervisee when she was not willing to meet certain expectations. As the reverse was not true for the supervisee, power was very unequal, despite the aim of supervision to be more empowering for all participants (ENB, 1997).

The multiple roles of the supervisor

The supervisor of midwives has several, concurrent, professional roles, as the work of supervision is carried out in conjunction with a midwifery post. The different requirements of each of these separate roles were potentially conflicting, as each carried with it a set of responsibilities and expectations. On some occasions the supervisor's personal ideology was in conflict with the needs of the supervisee. These issues were problematic because the subject of boundaries within the supervisory relationship was rarely discussed.

Managerial

Midwives consistently voiced anxieties about the maintenance of boundaries where the supervisor concurrently held a management position. This was even more problematic in trusts where the midwifery voice was weak, or absent, at senior management level.

The juggling of multiple loyalties has become an everyday experience for supervisors. Midwives interviewed described supervisors as accomplishing this with highly variable degrees of skill. Supervisors were often required to balance the needs of the employing organisation and the midwives they served within the supervisory relationship. They were expected to create and maintain an environment of confidentiality and support for the developing midwife, whilst simultaneously setting safe standards for practice, and assuring the delivery of a quality service to an ever more critical consumer and employing agency. The psychological pressures on individuals coping with competing demands, and the additional interpersonal conflicts generated from multiple role expectations, were seen as causing anxiety and stress. It was also widely acknowledged that constantly responding to, and prioritising the external demands of, the organisation, may require a degree of estrangement from, or denial of, the supervisor's own feelings.

In this study, some of the more junior midwives expressed a high degree of confidence in the ability of the supervisor to differentiate which role she was occupying and they trusted that this knowledge would be used to the benefit of the midwife:

> I would go to them for help and then hopefully they would be able to tell me whether it was a supervisory or a management issue.
> (F grade site one)

Interestingly, however, some of the student midwives appeared less trusting on this point:

> The midwifery managers are the gatekeepers into the profession in terms of getting jobs so you have to be careful and sometimes you might have to suck up to them a bit. (Senior midwifery student site three)

The more experienced midwives interviewed expressed a range of views on this subject and this reflected both their previous experiences and their changing perceptions.

The issue of supervisory roles is made more complex because of midwives' different, and sometimes conflicting, expectations of supervisors. Midwives certainly wanted support and an accessible supervisor with whom they could discuss, in confidence, issues which they might not wish to raise with their manager. At the same time, they wanted a supervisor to be an advocate for them; one whose words carried 'clout' in wider circles, particularly where the subject of resources was concerned. Whilst a non-manager was likely to be seen as more trustworthy in terms of support and confidentiality, she usually lacked the organisational power to act as an effective advocate for midwives.

Some units in the study tried to circumnavigate this problem by 'cross-supervision': ensuring that a supervisory case-load did not include those midwives for whom the supervisor was a direct line manager. Separating the roles in this way was commonly seen as a way of lessening prejudice and also of making available an 'uncontaminated' support system in cases where a midwife was under investigation, or perhaps facing disciplinary proceedings. It should not be necessarily assumed, however, that such a separation meant that any greater understanding of the underlying conflict had occurred.

A number of the supervisors interviewed appeared to be rather unclear in differentiating some aspects of their role and, although this was rarely admitted to as being problematic, it clearly affected the availability and calibre of support available to midwives.

Leadership

Many respondents linked leadership firmly and positively with supervision. The attributes required by the supervisor as leader on site two, for example, suggested an inclination toward a more equitable and interactive relationship. The commentaries from a range of respondents demonstrated that this required a constant shifting of viewpoint as information was received, exchanged and challenged. This attentive listening, and modifying of position, was in contrast to the management viewpoint, so evident on site three, which prioritised allegiance to the organisation over the need to model effective midwifery leadership.

Whilst respondents generally made a very strong association between leadership and supervision, not all supervisors were aware of this, nor were they sufficiently prepared to discharge this responsibility wisely and creatively. The issue of whether supervisors would be 'active advocates' and not merely 'good listeners', appeared troublesome for midwives of all grades, including LSA officers.

Underlying the various qualities of leadership is the fundamental issue of trust. The following quotations from midwives on site two demonstrate ways in which trust was nurtured by supervisors and the subsequent influence this had on the relationship between midwife and supervisor:

One of the important things in my relationship with my supervisor is the trust between us... I know X would trust me to know that if I've made a mistake... I'm no fool... we both know I won't make that mistake again. There was an incident once where... when I did go of my own accord to see her she said that she hadn't asked me to come because she knew me well enough to know I'd have realised my [drug] error... so we didn't need to have a discussion about it. That to me is wisdom... but more importantly to me, it's also about not abusing your position. That kind of leadership is really inspiring... it makes you want to try harder... it also makes me realise that it's something we all do together... it's not about the supervisor doing it for me – she can only put the tracks down. (F grade site two)

I trust her because I know where she's coming from and I respect her views... She's interested in me too... it means she can criticise me and offer me help without me falling apart or feeling like a complete failure... But then she's a very special woman... she's got a quiet kind of authority... I could never, ever imagine her losing her head. (E grade site two)

It is of note that these respondents fundamentally wanted the same things from supervision as respondents on other sites. Their experience of supervision, however, was such that they felt able to accept criticism constructively and that they appeared to be less vulnerable to the negative aspects of the wider culture of midwifery than were other respondents. It was also apparent that a number of supervisors on site two were actively building upon this basis of trust and that a shared philosophy of supervision was being developed and put into practice. This required great self-awareness and skill on the part of the supervisors. It also required that they often worked against the grain of the traditional culture of midwifery, but it provided powerful role models and an alternative set of values.

I feel very strongly about not creating a dependent relationship... I don't want them to be dependent on me. I'd like all of them to be able to challenge with confidence, to challenge the structure, to challenge me... I hope I show them that we can have meaningful discussions about practice issues and challenge each other respectfully... I've noticed they are often embarrassed by my approach initially, but then it gradually becomes a shared philosophy so that we all become accustomed to being challenged and being accountable... it becomes the normal thing to do... I think good supervision is tied up very closely with good leadership... anyone can carry a title and not be at all visible themselves but you can still see results in the development of the midwives... I really don't want midwives to look on me as just someone to go to because there's a problem... I really don't want to be seen as a fix-it-up person...

Another thing which I have learned through my role as a tutor is to tolerate criticism... to be able to apologise and tell them why I made certain decisions. (Clinical lecturer/supervisor site two)

... and it wasn't that she was outstandingly knowledgeable nor particularly eloquent even... It was her humility that was impressive; that and her humour and her ability to relate to you... but also to take you seriously when it was appropriate... That honesty and humility really impressed me. (E grade site two)

The two passages above beautifully illustrate many of the important features of the supervisee–supervisor relationship wherein the qualities of leadership are clearly in evidence. They support the principles of partnership and collaboration, rather than any desire to control or subvert the relationship. In so doing they truly empower. The parallels between the supervisory relationship and the relationship of midwife and client are very clear.

It is, however, difficult to separate the issues of authority and leadership within the supervisory relationship from the issues of location and distribution of power within the employing organisation. Supervisors who were not managers, or whose positions were dominated by more powerful general managers, might have considerable personal authority, but no direct access to resources nor to the powerholders. Supervisors who were managers often had certain institutional loyalties and these frequently conflicted with the personal and professional aspirations they held as supervisors.

The commitment which supervisors, as managers, gave to the ideologies of their employing organisations greatly influenced the quality and direction of their leadership and this consequently affected their ability to act as advocates for the midwives they supervised.

Mechanisms of control

The act of suspension and the function of discipline

The issue of suspension demonstrated the extent to which the supervisory and management roles were entwined. There are two different routes though which a midwife may be suspended: by her employer, in which case she is suspended from duty; or by the authority of an LSA officer, whereby she is suspended from practice. Thus a manager, who may or may not be a supervisor (or even a midwife), may suspend an employee from work. Suspension from practice was an unusual event: it occurred four times in England in 1996, and was encountered in this study only once. Suspension from duty, however, occurred more frequently.

Respondents used the word 'suspension' indiscriminately; many thought that supervisors could 'suspend' a midwife. Furthermore, very few respondents realised that a manager was not required to have the consent of the supervisor in order to suspend a midwife from duty; indeed the research team were made aware of a number of instances where supervisors were not even informed when this action was taken. Further difficulties were apparent in cases where management decided to pursue disciplinary action without soliciting the views of the supervisors. This occurred whenever managerial criteria for disciplinary action were different from the clinical practice criteria of a supervisor, as was frequently illustrated in the management of complaints from clients.

Some respondents suggested that, in contrast to their own position, the supervisor appeared to be insulated from the threat of suspension. One respondent went so far as to volunteer that this was possibly 'one of the few perks of the job'.

Midwives who had been suspended from either practice or duty, or who had been close to colleagues who had suffered this fate, often described the process in terms of death, disintegration and fragmentation.

> *Being suspended has been an absolute nightmare... the effect is indescribable... the shock... I'll never forget the feelings in my body... faint... sicky... sweaty... terrible headaches... and I couldn't focus or hear properly... one of the worst things is that you start to question everything about yourself – not just about*

being a midwife but... about everything. [Interview interrupted as respondent very distressed]... *the worst thing is the loneliness... just sitting around... all these years of working... how did I get to be such a bad person... and why did it need the mothers to complain – why didn't any of my colleagues tell me?* (F grade)

No matter how distant they were from the disciplinary mechanism, none of the supervisees interviewed suggested that suspension could ever be seen as anything other than an extremely negative and damaging event with long-term repercussions. This did not seem to be generally appreciated by supervisors. Some supervisors rationalised suspension from employment as being in the best interests of the midwife, even when it was acknowledged that the midwife's practice could not be faulted.

In the following passage, an LSA officer suggests that the impact of an adverse event upon a midwife could, in itself, make her unsafe to practise:

... as a supervisor and a manager you do have a responsibility to make sure that this girl is safe to continue practice because if you've got something really horrible hanging over you, you cannot always function as sanely as you would any other time... it could put you at risk yourself of doing something silly. I think we have a responsibility to that person to get them out of that. Some people find the easiest way is to suspend them from duty; others might send them off on holiday. (LSA officer)

The accounts of midwives who had been through the disciplinary process illustrated a number of worrying issues concerning the longer term impact of a disciplinary action.

G isn't working as a midwife anymore. She couldn't practise after that. Everything she did she had to ask someone to check... She feels she has been branded guilty. I doubt that she'll ever work as a midwife again. (G grade site three)

Some midwives, however, felt that the disciplinary aspect of supervision had an important function in the control of midwives:

I think the punitive side of supervision is a good thing... we've got to toe the line. (F grade).

Just as some respondents saw the value of supervision as being mainly for their colleagues rather than for themselves, so too was this issue of control through discipline thought to be 'a good thing' for others, rather than for the individual concerned.

The impact of disciplinary action upon a midwife was particularly devastating when she had openly admitted an error to her supervisor, only to have this admission responded to by disciplinary action through the management route. This made it even more difficult for midwives to distinguish between managerial and supervisory action because, in their minds, the process, and the outcome, of all disciplinary action was very similar.

> *Recently I had to write a statement because of a drug error which was minor and which I admitted responsibility for as soon as I realised. I am still bitter and very angry because it was handled so badly. Until then I had always been staunchly loyal, optimistic and very outgoing... but this has knocked the stool from under me... I have been given a verbal warning which will stay on my records for three years... There was no union representation because I had no idea this was going to happen. I was rung up on the ward and just asked to pop down for five minutes... The supervisor who is the HoM here has made light of it... but I'm completely gutted... I've dropped out of everything... I'm not sleeping... I'm terrified of making another mistake.* [Interview interrupted as respondent begins to sob uncontrollably] (F grade)

The decision taken by this supervisor in opting to deal with an admitted error in this way stands in sharp contrast with the account of a midwife on site two describing her supervisor's response to a similar scenario, where the admission of error was used to build both trust within the supervisory relationship, and confidence in the practitioner. The two accounts also illustrate the very different approaches to supervision to which midwives are currently exposed.

Where once disciplinary action concerned itself primarily with issues of clinical practice, in keeping with the need to maintain a corporate image, the wider gaze of the organisation seems now to be turning to what might be described as a policing of the more personal attributes of employees. These include aspects of the general 'deportment' of the individual, such as that of attitude.

The absence of a mechanism for appeal

One of the functions of supervision is that of protection of the public in terms of 'safety', and of the midwife in terms of ensuring that she is adequately supported, and is enabled to practise competently (ENB, 1997). What has not been addressed is the protection the midwife herself may need from supervision. A further problem, revealed by many of the accounts from respondents, is that within the current supervisory arrangements there is no formal structure for appeal with regard to local decision making. As this may also be the case for managerial decisions, it is perhaps small wonder that some respondents did report feeling vulnerable with respect to supervisory decisions which were made on their behalf, but in the absence of consultation. Mechanisms for challenging supervisory decisions are available to the midwife only in the rare event of a case being referred to the UKCC.

Some midwives were of the opinion that supervision was fundamentally flawed because of the absence of a mechanism for local appeal against supervisory decisions. Supervision, for these respondents, could not empower midwives because the midwife could not share power with the supervisor, nor challenge her decisions. It was also felt that the lack of such a mechanism created a situation where supervisors provided poor role models for clinical practice.

Incidences of midwives challenging decisions made by supervisors were very rare and were not reported at all where disciplinary action had been taken. Several respondents reported that, having been found deficient in some way, a period of supervised practice or retraining had been instituted without learning outcomes or evaluation. The experience was thus perceived as penitential rather than developmental.

Supervisors and supervision

The needs of the supervisor and her achievements

It is important to examine what supervisors see as their needs if they are to meet the needs of midwives. This leads to further issues of whether there are limits to the support supervisors can be expected to offer, and, perhaps more importantly, whether it is realistic to increase the scope of supervision without the infrastructure to identify and rectify the current failings and omissions.

> *I think supervisors in midwifery have to carry too much responsibility and there doesn't seem to be much support available for them... I'd hate to see midwifery going the same way as some of those ruthless American companies... but more and more I see that's the way it's going... with supervisors having to sift out the dead wood and that's just not fair on them... We have to learn to tolerate and learn to accept a certain amount of imperfection; it's exhausting and unreal, all of this striving to be perfect and getting ahead all the time!* (Senior midwifery student site two)

The support available to supervisors themselves varied greatly:

> *... our local supervising authority officer is excellent... she is so supportive... she is very available and approachable.* (HoM site five)

> *As a supervisor I got no support... I was out on my own... I was supposed to be acting autonomously, but as far as I'm concerned that just meant I was abandoned.* (G grade, former supervisor)

> *I think what concerns me most of all at the moment is that there are no mechanisms to enable us as supervisors to off-load and it's obvious that is needed... at the moment it's almost as if confidentiality has to leak out because supervisors have so little support and are so stressed that they are just not able to contain confidential information; they have to off-load onto one another and they are off-loading highly confidential information. I have to say that this confidentiality problem is not just a supervisor's problem though – it's a bigger midwifery problem that had never been addressed but that in itself suggests a serious professional deficit.* (LSA officer)

The above quotation from an LSA officer, who is in a position to take an overview of the situation, raises issues which are of great concern for supervisors, and for the wider culture of midwifery.

The needs of supervisors in situations of change were of particular significance on site five. This was because the supervisory philosophy held that a flattening of hierarchies and a devolution of power was important to all midwives.

> Interviewer: *Can you tell me a bit more about this issue of respect?*

Supervisors have to earn it by working very hard and doing something for the midwives. They have a difficult job sometimes because in this worrying environment there are always lots of things going on... there is still a lot of opposition to change despite the fact that there has been so much of it... sometimes the midwives' opposition is illogical... they don't think things through. So for supervisors to hold all that resistance and fear is a big job. (E grade site five)

Supervisors were very aware of the issue of resources in terms of what could be offered within the present structure of supervision. For many, this primarily concerned the allocation of time and its economic implications. Some midwives were of the opinion that supervision should be funded; that it should not be another (unpaid) role on top of a full time post.

A number of supervisors described the similarity between their own needs for good supervision, and those of their supervisees:

Interviewer: *What might good supervision for yourself actually look like?*

Well, it's probably exactly what I want to be able to give to the midwives and I can't – things like dedicated time when I know I'm going to be available for them, a relationship where we can both feel OK about giving and receiving feedback, someone for support... that kind of thing. (G grade supervisor)

Supervisors, like midwives, also operated within the changing NHS culture where rising litigation costs and the need to keep customers satisfied increasingly directs clinical practice. In this environment, the 'fear factor' was seen by many respondents as a major barrier to the further development of both supervision and of professional development.

There is clearly considerable potential for mismatch between the perceptions of those giving, and those receiving, a service. The lead supervisor on site five had clearly achieved much in enabling midwives to clarify key issues. The open and diverse viewpoints from which respondents described problems, and the expectations they had of resolving these, testified to real changes in the orientation of supervision on this site. These very changes, however, only served to add to the pressures upon the supervisors.

If the needs of supervisors are not addressed, there is a real risk of making supervision the dumping ground for midwives' unrealised fantasies which, when not met, contribute to a lowering of morale. Inappropriate expectations also encourage a 'shopping list' mentality, where both midwives and mothers demand what is simply not available, especially within the present economic climate and structure of the NHS.

References

Belenky, M.F., Clinchy, B.Mc., Goldberger, N.R., Tarule, J.M. (1986). *Women's Ways of Knowing: The Development of Self, Voice and Mind*. New York: Basic Books.

ENB. (1997). *Preparation of Supervisors of Midwives: an open learning programme*. London: ENB.

Fanon, F. (1963). *The Wretched of the Earth*. New York: Grove Press.

Glaser, B., Strauss, B. (1967). *The Discovery of Grounded Theory*. Chicago: Aldine.

Kirkham, M. (1999). 'The culture of midwifery in the NHS in England'. *Journal of Advanced Nursing*, Vol. 30, No. 3.

Leap, N. (1997). 'Making sense of "horizontal violence" in midwifery'. *British Journal of Midwifery*, Vol. 5, No.11, p. 689.

Royal College of Midwives. (1996). *In Place of Fear: Recognising and confronting the problem of bullying in midwifery*. London: RCM.

Stapleton, H., Duerden, J., Kirkham, M. (1998). *Evaluation of the Impact of the Supervision of Midwives on Professional Practice and the Quality of Midwifery Care*. London: ENB.

Strauss, A., Corbin, J. (1990). *Basics of Qualitative Research: Grounded Theory Procedures and Techniques*. London: Sage.

Helen Stapleton • Jean Duerden • Mavis Kirkham

Implications of
Current Supervision
for Midwifery Practice and Education

RESEARCH AND AUDIT

The supervision of midwives can only be justified by its contribution to the practice of midwifery. Yet, the contribution of supervision to practice is facilitative and thus operates at one remove from the clinical situation. Supervision is therefore to be judged in terms of its impact upon the practice of the midwives who actually care for childbearing families. Clearly, many other factors affect the practice of midwives and in turn interact with the use the midwife makes of her supervision.

Assessing the quality of midwifery care is a complex undertaking (Audit Commission, 1997). This study (see Chapters 2 and 3 and Stapleton, Duerden and Kirkham, 1998) did not aim to assess systematically the quality of midwifery care on the sites researched, though insights were gained and data from midwives were triangulated with data from focus groups with mothers.

The general impact of supervision

The midwives interviewed reported that supervision did have an impact upon their practice, particularly on the way in which they approached and coped with their work. This impact could be positive or negative. Comments ranged from 'supervision increases my energy and attention to my work', to 'it makes me feel drained, despondent and victimised'. Midwives also described how the impact of supervision on them, in turn, impacted upon their clients: 'I feel happier and so the women in my care feel happier'. Or, 'I feel despondent and depressed; this has a bad effect on the women who also then become ineffectual and don't achieve their full potential'. In the full report (Stapleton, Duerden and Kirkham, 1998) midwives' views on the impact of supervision on their practice are explored in detail using personal construct theory (Kelly, 1955).

Whilst midwives felt that supervision did influence their practice, the extent to which they could maximise that influence was limited by their ignorance of supervision. There are clear implications here for midwifery education. As the education of supervisors has been greatly helped by ENB publications (ENB, 1992 and 1997), a similar publication on supervision for students and midwives may be helpful here and has since been published (ENB, 1999).

Midwives identified a great need for support from supervision. Their ignorance of supervision, however, meant that some of their support needs were outside the remit of supervision and the rest were often given as a long list of needs, rather than being tailored in any way towards what supervisors could realistically provide. This suggests that a great many midwives had not learned about the real function or purpose of supervision during the process of being supervised. Nor had they received help in defining and focusing their needs so that they could find ways to ensure these needs were met either within, or outside of, the supervisory environment. This suggests a need for supervisors to gain the skills to facilitate such focusing and personal planning.

The local impact of differing approaches

It was clear from all the sites studied that supervision was closely linked with practice, though this was complicated by the tendency for facilitative supervisors to also be facilitative managers. When asked to describe the model of supervision operating locally, respondents either referred to their current supervisory relationship, or made statements about future ideals:

In some units I would say there is now a model where the supervision could be described as proactive, as being caring and supportive, but where it also aims to tackle the problems. (LSA officer site five)

If I were to design a model of supervision, I would want a relationship where there was respect for each other – personal as well as professional respect. I'd want it to be supportive, to be able to handle criticism but in a constructive way – not make me feel that I have done something wrong. (F grade site three)

The model of supervision here I'd say was good in that it does seem to help us to do our work better... I think both the supervisors here do work hard to see the positive side of things and they do praise us when things have been done well. (E grade site two)

A model of supervision?... I suppose I think that if I like someone then it's more likely that I'll be able to take criticism – I'll see it as a healthy exchange... and I'd want to be able to feed back to the supervisor... I'd expect her to be able to justify her actions... I would find it extremely difficult to accept a supervisor I didn't like as a person. (G grade site one)

A number of supervisors did appear to have taken the lead from the recommendations of the ENB in moving away from an inspectoral role toward developing a much broader remit for supervision. Such initiatives, however, tended to be associated with the personal style and philosophy of an individual supervisor and, as such, remained at a local, rather than a national, level of application. Site two was unusual in that it demonstrated evidence of power and authority being mutually and amicably shared between the supervisors at the DGH and their supervisees. The research team could find little evidence, however, of what might be described as a coherent model of supervision on any of the sites visited. This may be because the recent changes to supervision need more time to be absorbed and refined to suit local needs, or because the process of supervision does not conform to this descriptive framework.

The supervisory relationship

The supervisory relationship began as one controlling midwives and it has proved hard to transform this into an empowering relationship. A relic of that earlier relationship is the issue raised by a number of midwives on different sites that 'there is no appeal' against supervisory decisions, short of formal disciplinary action. This situation clearly works against openness, trust, negotiation and empowerment for the midwife and needs to be addressed.

To work towards empowerment in supervision is to work against the status quo, mutual expectations and complex defence reactions. Nevertheless, if midwives are to turn around their basic working relationships to be enabling for clients, midwives themselves need enabling supervision. Those who have experienced this find it strengthening, supportive and inspiring. The reduction in the ratio of midwives per supervisor could provide the opportunity and the necessity to improve and to define the nature of the supervisory relationship. This study identified key issues in the supervisory relationship and found great differences between sites.

The long-standing impact of supervision

The impact of supervision can be for good or ill, and that effect is likely to be long-lasting. The long-term good effects of supervision were vividly described by midwives:

I was involved in an incident which was very, very distressing... but I was supported so wonderfully by the supervisors and felt very cared for. That support was demonstrated for me... things like being given a lighter case-load for a bit and getting a hug from my supervisor and being told not to feel the blame. It's so different now. (G grade community midwife site two)

I was involved in a dreadful case... I went to see my supervisor... and we went through the notes together... it was very beneficial... I think it stopped me from really falling apart... just knowing that someone was there and they weren't blaming you or saying things about you behind your back. (E grade site two)

Such supervision was able to inspire and motivate midwives:

I'm not saying we haven't got problems... but she gives you the feeling it's possible to sort them out... everything cascades down from her. (F grade site five)

The empowering effect of such role modelling upon midwives was clear. Midwives were also aware of learning specific skills from this role modelling:

She has a way of being able to put everything into perspective... she always emphasises the positive and asks us what we can learn from a situation. (F grade site four)

A further important factor is the invisible nature of good supervision which can prevent a difficult situation from having a damaging effect upon midwives. A newly qualified supervisor on site one spoke of:

... accumulated wisdom... and collective experience and authority... really show... it probably prevents a lot of mistakes, together with 'gut intuition' based on long experience of supervision that is so valuable... I think you are most likely to see it operating in a crisis situation – but then if the supervisor really has it sussed you probably don't see it because it's so unobtrusive – there is no sign she's even been there – no trail of distraught midwives gossiping in corners – none of that sort of thing... They do it very naturally.

This is a shining example of the invisible excellence of supervisory practice which was providing a role model. It is difficult to monitor the absence of distraught midwives. Where they were present, however, that presence was very apparent.

The bad effects of supervision were also long-lasting, as was demonstrated on site four, where a number of midwives were still clearly traumatised by supervisory events which had happened some years previously. The value of debriefing traumatised clients is now being recognised and the same is likely to be true for midwives. Judging by the frequency of need encountered in this study, and the fact that such damage does not go away but continues to be acted out through defence mechanisms which limit individuals and their practice, debriefing is very important. This should be a key supervisory skill, or one which supervisors can access for midwives, otherwise individuals become increasingly scarred.

An issue frequently cited as traumatic supervision was the effect of a 'betrayal' of confidence. Midwives saw the betrayal of confidence as making them feel 'insecure'; as completely undermining their confidence in their supervisor and as ultimately affecting their self-confidence and their confidence in colleagues. Midwives who had the experience of confidence betrayed tended to withdraw and become defensive and muted. The defensive reactions resulting from such experiences could be damaging for both midwives and clients. However, the issue of confidentiality is complex, as was demonstrated on site one, where the keeping of confidentiality around an individual investigation led other midwives to feel anxious and threatened, and, as one respondent commented, 'then the women pick up our anxieties' (F grade site one). This study clearly demonstrated the common derivation of the words confidence and confidentiality!

Supervisors themselves spoke of needing support in stressful situations concerning confidentiality. Several stated that, 'There is no place for us to off-load any of it' (G grade supervisor site one).

Clearly, this is not a situation which can be sustained, so the maintenance of confidentiality also implies attention to the needs of the supervisor. The supervisor's situation is often extremely difficult, however, especially when she is judged on the revelation of one event which actually occurs in the context of many other events, all of which are confidential. The whole issue of confidentiality in supervision is highly complex. The supervisor must balance the needs of individuals and the collective body of midwives, as well as taking into account the other 'hats' she may wear, in addition to that of supervisor. This area is deserving of professional debate.

Vulnerability

Midwives appeared to feel vulnerable in the face of pressures from many directions and such pressures were often internalised, as was demonstrated throughout this study. Traditionally, supervision was seen by many midwives as a potential threat. When attempts were made to remove that threat, many midwives continued to experience a corrosive level of self-doubt and to empathise with threatened colleagues even where that empathy was completely inappropriate.

As midwifery practice changes, new areas of vulnerability are revealed. Traditionally, many of the more difficult relationships for midwives were those with colleagues outside the profession. On the occasions where midwife colleagues were perceived as deviant, however, there was evidence of these individuals being subjected to 'horizontal violence', from their peers or those very slightly senior to them, by way of punishment. The changing organisation of midwifery care, and the proliferation of pilot schemes in team midwifery and caseholding, have created new areas of vulnerability in relationships between midwives. In the evaluations of pilot midwifery projects it was common to find tensions between midwives in the team, and those working more traditionally (McCourt and Page, 1996). Accusations of 'elitism' and of having a 'cushy number' were also made by midwives in this study against colleagues working in different ways. This was particularly the case on sites where innovative midwifery projects were in evidence and must, therefore, be considered alongside the varying degrees of tension between hospital and community midwives. Newly qualified supervisors also spoke of tensions with colleagues and 'old style' supervisors. If midwifery is to progress in the direction suggested by *Changing Childbirth* (Department of Health, 1993), however, supervisors must be equipped to cope with these new vulnerabilities so that they, in turn, can help midwives to cope with them.

The exception to the general pattern of discomfort with new patterns of working was outside the NHS, where different working patterns were the norm rather than the exception, and respondents did not appear to feel threatened in the same way:

I think it's true to say that difference is seen as stimulating – it's well tolerated, it's not greeted with fear or anxiety... we don't hold a unified view of the world of pregnancy and birthing... or of the way midwives should do things... there are a lot of common views... Midwives all over the world do things differently... you can't expect one unified way of working... it's a false security to expect it... we all have very different styles... We do trust each other enough to say we don't understand something or to ask advice. (Self-employed midwife site six)

These respondents were also more inclined to express their vulnerability to one another and to expect to be supported in so doing:

I think a key issue for us is that since we've been in a group practice – the guiding/counsellor/friend aspect of supervision has been completely taken care of amongst ourselves... If we need support we turn to each other... our first point of reference would always be to each other. (Self-employed midwife site six)

Perhaps it is to be expected that where midwives are autonomous and confident they use midwifery supervision less. It may be the case that a really long-term aim of supervision is to render supervision, in its current state, unnecessary. As the original, socially controlling, aims of supervision are no longer needed, so the current enabling aims may be less needed at a future time when midwives are enabled to access other sources of support. Meanwhile, despite the institutional and personal constraints, supervision works towards that end.

Different areas of midwifery bring different vulnerabilities, as a midwife lecturer on site three observed:

I have attempted to see my supervisor twice, but have been unsuccessful. She made the comment that it wasn't needed: 'you're safe', but I feel I am very vulnerable ...

This raises the issue of how far supervisors are equipped to help midwives cope with their vulnerabilities when they are outside the mainstream. Similar descriptions of vulnerability came from agency and bank midwives, who also made it clear that no one was taking the role of supporter and advocate for them.

Supervisors are vulnerable too, and, in situations of threat from general management, midwives were aware of this:

> *Yesterday I saw one of the supervisors crying... it was after the manager had been to see her... to see her so unsupported and vulnerable makes me feel more vulnerable but quite happy because at least I know I'm not alone in this.* (E grade, recently disciplined)

Sadly, these two respondents are no less vulnerable because their position is shared. Midwives from across a spectrum of grades expressed feelings about the vulnerability of supervisors:

> *... you've also got to think of the poor supervisors taking all this on board – who do they go to when they're in trouble? They must need someone to go to in some situations... like if the midwife tells them something which is really not their problem to deal with... or which is really upsetting... I know it's all meant to be confidential but there must be some things they need to get advice on and to share with somebody?* (Newly qualified E grade site five)

Supervisors themselves occasionally voiced feelings of vulnerability, often in relation to specific events, such as the transition from midwife to supervisor. Supervisors were likely to feel isolated as well as vulnerable and for some there were no formal structures in place for their own supervision. Thus, not only did these supervisors have no supervisory setting in which to express their vulnerability, but they also lacked role models in their own supervision for providing this service for their supervisees.

Admitting to, and coping with, vulnerability is difficult in a culture where midwives are socialised to battle on and not admit to problems. Some supervisors offered midwives a safe opportunity to reflect on and learn from situations which made them feel vulnerable. In some of the sites studied, supervision also enabled midwives to access more specialist support services, such as clinical supervision.

Reflecting upon their vulnerability in a safe setting can equip midwives to give empathetic care to their vulnerable clients. Denial of vulnerability, or the masking of this by defence mechanisms, cannot help midwives to give good care. This is one of the many areas in which midwives felt that:

as midwifery practice changes, so must the role of the supervisor as there is more demand for advocacy. If midwives put themselves on the line for women, so must supervisors put themselves on the line for midwives. (Midwife, site five audit interview)

Dependency

There were many examples of supervision which fostered dependency from supervisees. Midwives and supervisors colluded in this, although some midwives expressed unease about it. This is not surprising from either side in view of our history, but it perpetuates the worst side of that history, i.e. the ongoing disempowerment of midwives and women and their powerless collusion with this process.

The fostering of dependence in the supervisory relationship falls into two categories. Firstly, there were examples of supervisors' need to control midwives and, in so doing, to inhibit their professional autonomy. A remark from a supervisor such as 'you're right to feel scared' (E grade site one) clearly falls into this category. Dependency was also encouraged on occasions when the supervisor inappropriately intervened in a situation:

[the supervisor] *insisted on being involved even though it had nothing to do with her... she made me update her every day... I felt like she'd taken over.* (G grade community midwife site one)

Paradoxically, it was also a feature in situations where supervisors refused to become involved in disputes between midwives, as this perpetuated a pattern of helplessness with respect to conflict resolution:

... if that situation had been nipped in the bud when they had gone to see the supervisor here... if she had done something, it would have been different... Nobody was really helped... all she was doing was playing the midwives off against one another and getting a quick get out for herself... the easy way out. (G grade community midwife site five)

Secondly, there were examples of inappropriate 'caring' for the midwife by the supervisor: a 'nannying' which does not fit with the professional status of either midwives or supervisors. The supervisor reminding the midwife of her need for statutory updating, for example, as distinct from the discussion of how to make best use of such updating for professional development, falls into this category. It could also be argued that the checking of intention to practise forms by supervisors, whilst useful in the days when many midwives were illiterate, could now be seen as inappropriate nannying. This is not to say that supervisors do not need to be notified of midwives practising in their area, but the checking of their ability to correctly complete and sign these forms uses vast amounts of supervisors' time and, furthermore, could be seen as encouraging careless record keeping. Nannying is, of course accepted by some midwives although it is rather alarming to hear a midwife say of a supervisor that 'she is obligated to look after me' (G grade site five) in this way.

Many supervisors were, however, working hard to facilitate midwives' autonomy although this was not always easy as 'they expect you to do everything for them... but I just put that right back to them... they can organise that for themselves'. (G grade supervisor site five). Very occasionally, supervisors were explicit about 'not creating a dependent relationship... I'd like them all to be able to challenge with confidence, to challenge the structure, to challenge me...' (Supervisor, site two). This particular supervisor went on to explain how she worked towards this by challenging her supervisees, '... but I do it quietly, and confidentially and privately, so it's not a public thing'. The supervisors in the DGH on site two had clearly progressed a long way in this direction and had empowered midwives to feel in control of their work situation and to have respect for the limitations of their supervisors:

> ... she shouldn't be lumbered with our bright ideas unless they are really going to benefit the unit... and it's up to us to prove that... to help her make a case for management to consider it. We should be blowing our own noses, not expecting her to do it. (E grade site two)

Examining dependency in supervision inevitably raises wider issues of dependency both within the NHS and in society. There is a real sense in which the 1902 Midwives Act made midwifery dependent upon medicine, and the shadow of that dependency blends with the traditionally dependent position of women in our society. We are now, however, in a very different social climate where dependence takes new forms. The market economy has greatly emphasised the role of the consumer in recent years. Whilst the consumer may have been given rights and entitlements, and encouraged to exercise choice, it is fundamentally a passive role. The data generated by the survey contained a number of examples of midwives' passive expectancy with regard to their supervisor. This is certainly not empowering and merits wider debate.

Resistance to change

There is a natural human tendency to stick with what is known and familiar, and the history of midwifery reinforces this. It is not surprising that new supervisors tend to stick to the clearly defined, and historically secure, ground of inspection and review. They appeared to be more secure in asking specific things of midwives than in coping with the complex uncertainties of facilitation and empowerment. Excellent mentorship could facilitate exceptions to this. The power of custom, especially where reinforced by mentorship, was evident even when this was in a very different direction from the emphasis in the taught course, which is upon the enabling aspect of supervision. The mentor clearly occupied a powerful position in the education and subsequent practice of supervisors. Mentorship for the new supervisors' course was inevitably drawn from amongst those supervisors who had not themselves undertaken this course. To some extent, this acted as a brake upon the aims of the course to fundamentally change the emphasis of supervision. At the time of writing, this is beginning to change as supervisors prepared through the new path attain the seniority to become mentors themselves. This was not the case at the time of data collection.

The influence of mentorship also serves to emphasise the importance of using this facility to widen the network of resources available to a supervisor. In this context, the gains of having a good mentor who is not already known to the student supervisor, e.g. from another unit, may well outweigh the inconvenience of distance. It can be argued that the conservative effect of mentorship is

> *a bit like any other theory–practice gap... you teach them one thing in the classroom and they go and see the opposite happening on the ward.* (midwife lecturer site two)

This raises the universal problem of how practice can ever be changed. If the emphasis of supervision is on positive change, which is the explicit aim of the new open learning programme, then careful attention needs to be paid to the selection and training of mentors so that they work in the same direction. Mentorship training using the 1997 ENB open learning programme is thus likely to improve the training of supervisors.

It is ironic that supervisory and mentorship relationships tend to lack defined boundaries. Mentorship which encourages boundaries to be clearly defined is essential for both the supervisor and the supervisee. A task without end cannot be done, let alone done well, and if the new supervisor is not taught how to establish the limits of her role and her skills in specific situations, she will also be unable to refer midwives elsewhere for support and advice when this is appropriate. Skill in establishing and acknowledging boundaries was seen to be a key factor in giving supervisors the security to cope with change.

Exploring the issue of boundaries is an important step towards role definition, which in turn can bring into clearer focus what supervisors actually do. Such work would create greater openness rather than the 'doing good by stealth' which is so much a part of both supervision and midwifery. While this may achieve immediate objectives, it models manipulation rather than negotiation, and as such cannot empower or increase confidence.

It is clearly essential that supervisors are aware of, and develop skill in coping with, resistance to change and tendencies towards being manipulative, both in themselves and in their supervisees. Confidence and confidentiality are the foundations for such work. The analysis from site five demonstrates a key point in the development of an enabling model of supervision: whereby discord has to be voiced, rather than suppressed, before midwives can work together towards the future. An E grade midwife on site five spoke perceptively about using vulnerability to help achieve this:

> ... there has to be something to be gained by bringing vulnerability into the workplace and setting aside time for people to say how they feel and until that happens there isn't going to be any fundamental change in midwifery – it's going to remain stuck at the Laura Ashley wallpapering over the cracks.

It must be stressed that the quality of supervision is a factor quite separate from the supervisory case-load. Ironically, it was on site two, where the supervisory case-load was largest, that midwives were most satisfied with their supervision. The strong ethic of fostering independence possibly enabled those supervisors to cope with their large case-loads; they also achieved the most frequent contact between supervisors and supervisees of all the NHS sites studied. This is not to suggest that the supervisory case-load should not be decreased, but to stress that this will only achieve the level of supervision which enables good practice where attention is specifically given to the quality of the supervisory relationship and its clinical aims.

Changing the culture of supervision

Supervision can be of great help to midwives in fostering their abilities to practice autonomously. The audit showed that 20 per cent of last supervisory contacts had been initiated by the midwife seeking professional advice from her supervisor. This could be interpreted as encouraging and may provide a foundation upon which to build.

Choice of supervisor

If supervision is to serve midwives' needs and help them to work towards meeting their own needs, there is a need for midwives to feel more control within the supervisory relationship. A step towards this would be for midwives to choose their supervisor. Most midwives interviewed wanted this. Such choice would give the midwife control in relation to the dilemma of whether or not to be supervised by her manager. It should also prove a useful first step towards a relationship of trust and equality. Encouraging choice of supervisor might also help with the social difficulties and inhibitions many midwives felt around changing their supervisor, despite the fact that it was organisationally possible to do so.

Choice of supervisor would need to be based upon knowledge and many issues need to be specifically examined. These issues include whether midwives should just make an initial choice, or should exercise this choice at regular intervals and what information should be provided to midwives as a basis for choice. This latter point raises for debate the topic of audit of supervision and to whom such audit results should be made available. Debate on these issues would, in itself, be one step towards professional empowerment. Such debate could be initiated by a sensitive publication for midwives from the ENB.

Choice for supervisors was also an issue. Many supervisors were reported to have a small degree of informal choice of supervisees in some large units. Asking midwives to name two or three supervisors who would be acceptable to them would give both sides a degree of choice in large units. Choice will always be a problem in remote rural areas where there are few staff and only one supervisor. In such circumstances it is particularly important that supervisors are able to facilitate midwives in making the maximum use of all available means of gaining appropriate support. A senior midwifery student on site one suggested an area worth exploring:

> *You could set up a web page on the Internet and have a midwives'*
> *support group and then you wouldn't need supervisors for that*
> *so much.*

The logic which suggests that midwives choose their supervisor would also extend to a role for supervisees in monitoring and evaluating supervisory performance. This is likely to be empowering and educational for midwives. It could only be embarked upon, however, when midwives have considerably greater knowledge of supervision than the majority of those studied.

Supervisory meetings and empowerment

Midwives could also control the agenda of more supervisory meetings, rather than following a routine agenda set by the supervisor. Many midwives expressed a need for a supervisor to be 'someone... who I am free with... who is easy to talk to' (F grade site five). For many midwives, however, the supervisory review is still approached with feelings of apprehension: 'I don't know anything. What's she going to ask me?' (F grade site five). Midwives tended to see all interviews as tests, even when those interviewing went to great lengths to stress the informality and confidentiality of the occasion. The midwife last quoted went on to tell the interviewer that, before her supervisory review, she felt 'a bit like coming here to talk to you really!' Clearly, there is a need to proceed beyond such apprehensions and out of the habit of feeling tested and ignorant. Progress could probably be made by transferring control of the review to the supervisee. This has the added advantage of modelling such a transfer of control.

A number of respondents, including LSA officers, spoke of the unproven value of the supervisory review in its present form. Whilst supervisory reviews provided visible evidence of supervision and the majority of midwives in this study wanted supervision to continue, there was evidence that the general style of supervision currently offered was not necessarily what midwives wanted. A preference was expressed by some respondents for more frequent, informal, meetings, rather than what they felt to be the overly-structured nature of the annual supervisory review. There was a sense, however, that the very structure provided a supporting ritual which was particularly comforting for new supervisors. Whilst it permitted them to monitor their work more easily, it also had the potential to emphasise its inspecting, rather than empowering, aspects.

Twenty-four hour access to a supervisor was available in every trust and the vast majority of midwives interviewed stated that, in an emergency, they could access a supervisor. Considerable numbers of midwives did not see supervision as having any function outside of emergency situations, however. They tended to limit the usefulness of supervision to immediate problem solving and as affording them some protection from litigation. It was rare for supervision to be seen as providing opportunities for enhancing practice or as a vehicle aiding professional development. Educating midwives to see supervision in this light is clearly possible, but very difficult to achieve with the current constraints upon supervisors' time.

All of the issues surrounding the meetings between supervisors and supervisees highlight the difficulty of the supervisors' position. To provide enabling supervision, they must listen to midwives and accept that some of their current supervisory practice is not acceptable. This is not easy to do when midwives still demonstrate considerable ignorance about supervision and it falls to the supervisor, whose best efforts they may appear to be rejecting, to educate the midwives. Supervisors are thus in a vulnerable position, often with very little support for themselves.

Neither the observation of practice by supervisors, nor the checking of bags belonging to community midwives, helped midwives to see themselves as autonomous professionals with the confidence to empower others.

Enhancing midwives' confidence

Midwives gave examples of a number of ways in which their confidence was enhanced. Some of these were very simple and centred upon the midwife feeling valued.

> *It's quite inspirational when people appear interested in you... it spurs me on... I feel motivated.* (F grade site five)

Midwives were surprised and heartened at being praised by a supervisor. They never expected praise and many expected blame because this was their habitual experience, even when there was nothing to blame them for. In such a climate midwives did not expect support:

> *... to be quite honest I've never known it... I think it would be quite amazing to have professional support.* (F grade site four)

They did, however, express a great need for support. In such circumstances, the expression of praise and thanks can initially change the atmosphere and ultimately be a move towards changing the culture. The expression of praise where it is due does not require extensive psychotherapeutic training. It takes little time and makes midwives feel valued. This valuing should, in turn, reflect on the supervisor who may herself be the victim of this culture.

There are other simple techniques which can help to improve the atmosphere of supervision. One that seems appropriate, and which comes from a similar context, is that of 'equality of esteem'. This term was coined by Charlotte Williamson (1997) in the context of the liaison between service providers and service users in primary care. Whilst efforts to hold all parties in equal esteem will not dissolve power differences, they should lead to people being consciously treated as equals. This practice, in its giving and receiving, may help to dissolve some of the disabling expectations of blame which midwives carry with them in so many situations.

Behind the issue of blame lies the question of who is at fault and the need to cover oneself in the expectation of blame. In this environment, the 'fear factor' was seen by many respondents as a major barrier to progress in both supervision and professional development.

> *I don't know how we get around the fear factor of supervision... it would make my life as a supervisor so much easier if I didn't have to cope with that as well.* (G grade supervisor manager)

> Interviewer: *You said something about our relationships as midwives?*

We all work as individuals and there is this huge, scary thing about 'covering yourself'. It makes you choose carefully who you discuss things with... and there is also this very scary phrase that midwives repeat when they are scared of doing something. They say 'it's your registration you're risking' and that brings a lot of fear. You hear it repeated as students... and you hear it repeated to mothers when they do something the midwife or the doctor doesn't agree with. They say 'you're risking your baby' and then the mother gets very anxious and frightened...

Interviewer: *Any ideas as to what this fear is about?*

It's because of the UKCC, because you could be suspended and then removed from the register. (Senior midwifery student)

Within this culture, even professional regulation, originally sought by midwives to enhance professional confidence, is seen through a lens of vulnerability and fear. Some supervisors were able to help midwives in naming and examining fears, as was the case on site five, but such issues were generally avoided.

A number of midwives recounted how they conscientiously brought an error to the attention of the supervisor and suffered for so doing. Other midwives explained that they did not disclose errors for fear of what would happen to them. In such a climate of fear, professional development is inhibited. It is difficult to learn from one's mistakes if those mistakes cannot be openly admitted and, in such situations, any policy of risk management is fundamentally flawed. This can be dealt with positively in supervision:

You want a supervisor... who can say 'Well, with hindsight, maybe it would have been better to... but I understand the rationale for why you did it and let's learn from it'. I think all midwives – including supervisors – need to grow up a bit about making mistakes. (Self employed midwife site six)

Risk management, at the level of supervision or of trust management, is only as good as the reporting of critical incidents and this is likely to be impaired by a culture of blame and concealment. Some risk management documents have declarations such as:

The Trust Board have stated that no disciplinary action will result from reported incidents or mistakes which are admitted. Exceptions to this rule will include criminal or malicious activities.

This was not, however, the approach taken on any of the sites researched. The research team also came across circumstances which, in fact, were quite the reverse and where midwives still felt themselves to be blamed or stigmatised even when they had been cleared of any fault:

... even though it was proved in the end that I was faultless, at the time it was such a stigma that I couldn't even share it with my husband.

After a complaint had been made against a midwife, it was felt on some sites that:

The midwife is guilty until proved otherwise and even if you can prove otherwise she is still guilty, because the client is still unhappy. So you can't win. (G grade site 3)

This assumption of guilt on all sides is a factor in the culture of midwifery which impedes progress in supervisory relationships, and is also likely to impede innovations in clinical care.

Skills, relationships and attitudes

There are parallels between the skills valued in supervision and those which maternity service users valued in midwives caring for them. Highly developed and flexible skills in empathy and support were clearly seen by service users as important in clinical midwifery and by midwives as important in supervision.

The expectations midwives had of supervisors may be seen as demonstrating many assumptions about the innate talents or acquired skills of the midwives who take on the supervisory role. These expectations included skills in everyday use in supervision such as listening, facilitating decision making and advocacy as well as skills specific to particular situations such as debriefing and conflict resolution, together with overarching skills of leadership, empowerment and giving midwives a voice. All these skills were demonstrated by some of the supervisors in this study, and, where they were exercised, their influence upon supervisory relationships and the culture of midwifery was certainly positive. They also modelled change in relationships which midwives reported as having a positive effect upon their relationships with colleagues and clients. Such examples show that changing the culture of supervision can have a really positive effect upon the culture of midwifery. Yet expecting the body of supervisors to exhibit the skills of a small number of their outstanding colleagues is to expect achievements of supervisors which may be beyond their talents, their experience and their education.

It is important to acknowledge that many of the situations currently faced by supervisors demand a range of highly skilful responses which need to be learned and which may be very different from the role models which have influenced them. It is also necessary to challenge the presumption that midwives, as (predominantly) women who have chosen to work in a caring profession, are equipped with all the necessary attributes; that they do not need to actually learn to be compassionate, accepting, sensitive, open, non-judgmental, warm, honest or trustworthy. If these attributes are to be learnt, then attention must be given to providing a safe and appropriate learning environment.

Where supervision was perceived by midwives as empowering, professional developments, including changes in attitudes, were reported. This appears to be linked with the nature of the supervision and to supervisory relationships which were seen as trustworthy and which provided a firm foundation for professional growth. In these circumstances, midwives and supervisors were able to move away from the guilt and fear which inhibit growth. Where supervision was less of an influence and general management reinforced the midwifery culture of guilt and fear, 'attitude problems' were identified as a cause of concern.

The question of changing attitudes is clearly complex. The attitudes in midwives which were identified as needing to be changed often seemed to be defensive in origin, i.e. they had, at some point in that midwife's history, probably served a useful purpose. The confidence an individual needs to change outmoded attitudes is clearly lacking when that same individual feels threatened. Furthermore, the courage to undertake personal change of this dimension is unlikely to be generated through punitive supervision or management. This is clearly a complex and sensitive issue which merits further study as well as professional debate.

Any investigation of supervisory skills inevitably raises questions about the adequacy of current training and the fact that what can be reasonably expected of a supervisor, including the limitations of her role, has not yet been defined.

Trust and boundaries

Trust is a central issue in the supervisory relationship, just as it is in the midwife–client relationship. Confidentiality is essential for the building of trust. Beyond the basic issue of confidentiality, trust arises from knowledge of what can be expected within a relationship. An LSA officer had important thoughts on this subject:

> I'd really like to tease out this issue of what we mean by 'support'. I'd like it defining – because I think that until the supervisor knows what she means by support, and how she is going to provide that support, and what her own limits are, then the midwives don't know what is on offer and they are not going to trust it. (LSA officer)

Definitions, then, are crucial. Trust is linked with knowledge of what is possible and where the boundaries of the relationship lie. This is very different from the limitless, female, caring role. It is also different from the vast list of support needs midwives in this study requested of supervisors. It is important that midwifery, as a profession, acknowledges that supervisors cannot do everything. A role which is treated as a dump for a profession's woes can never be successfully filled. Supervisors need to be facilitated in modelling to midwives that they cannot provide everything and that boundaries have to be constantly negotiated if any task is to be done successfully.

Support needs and trust

Two conflicting discourses run throughout the data collected from midwives within the NHS. The first concerned midwives' need for support, as described in the audit and as a recurrent theme in the in-depth interviews. These were often presented as lists of needs rather than grouped to realistically fit possible sources of support. The second discourse concerned the issue of trust and the many ways in which midwives felt unable to trust supervisors, managers or colleagues. Past experience of confidence betrayed or horizontal violence experienced, seen in action against a colleague, or simply envisaged as logical within the culture of midwifery, served to undermine trust.

There is thus a real contradiction between the expressed need for support and the surrounding culture which undermines the trust which is needed before support can be accepted. It may be this very contradiction which led to midwives being muted in terms of developing their discourse on support beyond an unstructured list. On the other hand, it may have been the general feeling of powerlessness described by many midwives which, together with a culture where mutual support is largely lacking and role models for support are rare, prevented midwives from analysing their own support needs. Midwives in this study very rarely looked at their support needs in a way which could act as a first step towards planning how these needs could be met.

The inertia which resulted from this conflict and which prevented midwives from progressing towards the meeting of their support needs was not present outside the NHS. Non-NHS midwives planned and developed support structures for themselves and saw the support they gained from colleagues, clients and members of other professions as very important for their personal and professional development and well-being. They did not, therefore, express the support needs with regard to supervision that were expressed by NHS midwives. This may be because they have opted out of the NHS and its culture of midwifery or it may be that their very different models of midwifery practice give them much more opportunity to develop appropriate support networks.

In *Making sense of 'horizontal violence' in midwifery*, Leap (1997) is of the opinion that:

It is possible that the key to moving out of a midwifery culture where horizontal violence persists can be found in developing models of midwifery care that offer autonomous and positive interprofessional collaboration with ensuing increased self-esteem for midwives, and a breaking down of hierarchies.

She goes on to examine how, in Australia Brodie (1996) has shown that, where midwives work in ways that allow closer relationships with women, the needs of the women become paramount with a resulting lessening of allegiance to profession or employer. This lessening of restrictive allegiances allowed scope for the development of new support networks. This was probably also true of the non-NHS respondents in this study. Another trend, however, is also seen in Brodie's research, Henderson's (1997) research, and the present study. This showed very difficult relationships, resistance to change and high levels of horizontal violence between midwives working in traditional ways adjacent to schemes which allowed closer relationships between midwives and clients. Such change was clearly perceived as threatening to those not immediately involved in it. This might account for many supervisors' persistent lack of interest in non-NHS midwifery, as frequently reported by independent and privately employed midwives.

The threat of change experienced by midwives working alongside new models of clinical care, and the possibility of developing trusted support networks by those outside the traditional models and culture, add further dilemmas to the conflicting discourses on the need for support and the barriers to trust. There is a pressing need for professional debate on these issues as they block progress towards achieving the aims of *Changing Childbirth* (Department of Health 1993), as well as towards improving supervision.

Power and supervision

Clout

'Clout' was an important issue to a large number of the midwives on all the sites studied. Clout is defined as, 'a blow, power or influence, especially political' (Collins Dictionary, 1987). It is taken here to mean the power of the supervisor, usually in organisational terms, to act as an advocate for midwives and mothers. Managers were seen as having more clout than non-managers:

> *If you take the supervision completely out of management you are losing a lot of clout.* (LSA officer)

A non-manager supervisor on site four gave a very sad example of her unsuccessful efforts to arrange a programme of supervised practice for a midwife whom the trust weren't prepared to employ any longer as a midwife:

> *... It was dreadful realising I had no clout... that I was just a supervisor... She [the business manager] was the one with all the clout. Anyway the midwife went off sick and never came back... then the business manager left.* (G grade)

Sometimes midwifery managers' clout was reduced by the overarching power of general management:

> *The labour ward manager has no budgetary control and she just cannot get the message across to management that the situation is very, very serious.* (F grade site three)

Sometimes lack of clout was seen as due to inexperience as supervisors:

> *... all this inexperience means that none of them can stand up to management... they haven't got an ounce of clout in them.* (E grade site three)

In other instances, individual qualities were seen to enhance the clout of a supervisor and clearly these individual skills could also be used to enhance the degree of clout which goes with a management position.

The issue of clout raises two of the several, and potentially conflicting, roles within the 'community' (Mair, 1977) of roles which constitute supervision. The listening and counselling role of the supervisor is very different from that of the advocate who has the power to take organisational action:

> *The problem is that a person who is a good listener isn't necessarily a good negotiator... there's a good side to having supervisors who aren't managers, but there's also a bad side because they haven't got the clout.* (G grade site three)

> *Supervisors need to be good listeners and good observers... and they need to have quite a bit of diplomacy and assertiveness... you need to be able to see yourself as someone who could carry out an argument with the chief executive for example.* (LSA officer)

The link between clout and managerial position can create problems as the numbers of supervisors increase and midwives' expectations of supervisors rise accordingly. Many of the new supervisors were of clinical grades which could increase their empathy with clinical midwifery colleagues, yet this did not give them clout. There is a real tension between the leadership and the supportive aspects of supervision. If a supervisor is in a position to hold sufficient power to have a positive influence on behalf of midwifery in wider forums, this may well reduce her effectiveness in the friend and counsellor aspect of her role because of her identification with management in the eyes of midwives. As a manager, she will also have to balance the interests of the midwives with the interests of the trust.

The need for clout in supervision is made more acute by the recent reduction in the numbers of midwife managers as a result of management cuts over which midwives have had little control, and also because of moves to create structures which are less hierarchical and which give clinicians more autonomy. This flattening of management structures can be seen as increasing the importance of supervision (Warwick, 1996). Thomas and Mayes (1996) look at flattening managerial structures in the context of the need for professional leadership 'at clinical, Trust Board and purchasing authority level'. Henderson (1997) stresses the importance of managerial effectiveness for midwifery. She emphasises that without midwifery managers at a senior level where they can 'influence and participate in decisions about reshaping services with professionals, women and commissioning authorities', a quality maternity service may not be achieved. Issues of clout, supervision and management are clearly very closely linked.

The issue of clout is also linked with that of leadership. There is a need for professional debate as to how it may be possible for supervisors to become professional leaders without creating a new hierarchy within supervision. As the number of supervisors who are not managers grows, there is a need for debate and local planning on the issues of clout and leadership in supervision.

Clout is clearly necessary and attention needs to be paid to identifying, fostering and using it appropriately. There also needs to be close liaison between supervisors with differing areas of expertise. At present, there are conflicting messages, since the need for supervisors as leaders is stressed alongside the need for supervisors from clinical grades. The supervisors who were seen as leaders and excellent role models on site two, for example, demonstrated an equitable and interactive relationship with midwives. Midwives described how this required a constant shifting of viewpoint as information was received, exchanged and challenged. This attentive listening and adjusting of position is a key skill in midwifery and advocacy, and stands in contrast to mainstream management which prioritises allegiance to the organisation.

There is an extent to which the supervision of midwives has some clout, at least enough to guarantee its continued existence, because of its statutory nature. There is a dilemma, however, as supervision came into statute as a measure of discipline and control. The dilemma relates to the authority invested in the statutory element of midwifery supervision, yet as one respondent commented:

> *I am not comfortable with that being linked to discipline... but it is an issue we will have to resolve because increasingly nurses are arguing that although they safeguard practice through clinical supervision, at the end of the day, it hasn't got clout and it's the clout bit – and as the word suggests, linked very much to discipline – that is different with midwifery.* (Supervisor site two)

Standards, discipline and education

The monitoring and policing aspects of supervision reflect its origins and were important to the many midwives who derived security from this function with regard to others. Those who experienced supervisory investigations were marked by the experience. Where that process was experienced as positive, there was professional growth. Where it was experienced as negative, midwives felt punished and were often resentful.

Where a supervisor is concerned about the practice of a midwife, or if a critical incident has occurred which has highlighted the need for professional development, the supervisor is expected to direct that development. Considerable planning is required if the outcome is to be positive. Whether this is to be achieved by means of a programme of planned supervised practice or an educational programme, it must be designed to meet the identified needs of the midwife concerned. The creation of such programmes, the drawing up of mutually acceptable learning contracts, the establishment of learning outcomes and methods of assessing whether those learning outcomes have been achieved, are all areas requiring time and considerable educational skill. Most supervisors are not trained as teachers and are therefore likely to need access to educational support. Without clear planning and justification, programmes of supervised practice or theoretical education can be highly unsuitable, which is why they are so often seen by midwives as a 'punishment' or a 'penance' rather than an educational process. Clearly this must change.

There are particular problems in planning and providing programmes of supervised practice or theoretical training in such a way that midwives feel ownership of the educational process. Such issues of empowerment in education should reasonably be seen as the province of midwifery education. These issues are particularly sensitive where the problem is one of the attitude of the midwife rather than any deficiency in her clinical skills. In these circumstances, very sensitive and educationally sound help may be required.

A partnership between midwifery supervision and midwifery education is required, to support clinicians in producing midwifery practice of sustainable excellence.

Leadership

Clearly, the exercise of power, both within the supervisory relationship and by supervisors as the leaders or advocates for midwives, needs wider professional debate and strategic thought. It would be useful to explore the differences between key midwifery skills in clinical practice and in leadership and the skills valued in NHS management. This would give greater understanding of the way that, in professional and managerial contexts, midwifery leaders are constantly judged by two very different sets of standards. Since midwifery skills are centred on facilitating individual achievement, whether in birth or professional life, it could be that, if modern NHS management is to prove sustainable, skills could be mutually learned. Without such debate there is a danger that mixed messages to supervisors and midwives will lead to a degree of confusion which could dilute the very clout which midwives see as so necessary from supervision and professional leadership.

There is also a need for professional debate as to which areas of support lie within the supervisor's role, as supervisors will have both differing and complementary areas of skill. One support skill that supervisors must have, which links with acknowledging boundaries, is the ability to act as a conduit to other means of support. This is the equivalent of the clinical midwife's knowledge of support groups and ways in which mothers can access support for themselves. No midwife can know everything, but the more skilled will always know someone who does, (be that a self-help group, a counselling service or a therapist), or, if necessary, will be able to refer to a database or book. With increasing confidence, supervisors can act as guides towards many ways of gaining support, thus helping midwives, and making their own workload more manageable. The building of the networks supervisors need to achieve this could enhance their 'clout' in a wider context.

Conclusion

There are great complexities in transforming supervision into a well-developed, practical medium for enabling and supporting midwives. In this process there will be much discomfort as suppressed conflicts and problems come out into the open, but this is a necessary first step towards finding solutions. Midwives' needs from supervision, as expressed in this study, are very similar to clients' needs from their midwife, in 'seeking a service that is respectful, personalised and kind, which gives them control and makes them feel comfortable in the sense of being at ease in the environment of childbirth and having confidence in their care' (DoH, 1993). Throughout this study, it has been demonstrated that supervision should, and could, provide for midwives what *Changing Childbirth* (DoH, 1993) requires the midwife to provide for her clients. This 'midwifing the midwife' (Taylor, 1996), is highly skilled and sensitive work, especially when the wider setting is unsupportive. The support, supervision and education available to supervisors is therefore fundamental to good midwifery care.

References

Audit Commission. (1997). *First Class Delivery: Improving Maternity Services in England and Wales*. Abingdon: Audit Commission Publications.

Brodie, P. (1996). Being with women: The experience of Australian team midwives. Unpublished Masters thesis, University of Technology, Sydney, Australia.

Department of Health (1993). *Changing Childbirth*. London: HMSO.

ENB (1992). *Preparation of Supervisors of Midwives: An open learning programme*. London: ENB.

ENB (1997). *Preparation of Supervisors of Midwives: An open learning programme*. London: ENB.

ENB (1999). Supervision in Action. London: ENB.

Henderson, C. (1997). *'Changing Childbirth' and the West Midlands Region 1995-1996*. London: RCM.

Kelly, G. (1995). *The Psychology of Personal Constructs* (Vols 1 and 2). London: Routledge.

Leap, N. (1997). Making sense of 'horizontal violence' in midwifery. *British Journal of Midwifery* Vol.5, No.1, p. 689.

McCourt, C., Page, L. (1996). *Report on the evaluation of one to one midwifery*. London: Thames Valley University and the Hammersmith Hospital.

Mair, J.M.M. (1977). 'The Community of Self'. In: Bannister, D. (ed.) *New Perspectives in Personal Construct Psychology*. London: Academic Press.

Stapleton, H., Duerden, J., Kirkham, M. (1998). *Evaluation of the Impact of the Supervision of Midwives on Professional Practice and the Quality of Midwifery Care*. London: ENB.

Taylor, M. (1996). 'An ex-midwife's reflections on supervision from a pyschotherapeutic viewpoint'. In: Kirkham, M. (ed.) *Supervision of Midwives*. Hale: Books for Midwives Press.

Thomas, M., Mayes, G. (1996). 'The ENB perspective: Preparation of supervisors of midwives for their role'. In: Kirkham, M. (ed.) *Supervision of Midwives*. Hale: Books for Midwives Press.

Warwick, C. (1996). 'Supervision and practice change at Kings'. In Kirkham, M. (ed.) *Supervision of Midwives*. Hale: Books for Midwives Press.

Williamson, C. (1997). *Some General Principles on Partnership*. Seminar proceedings, London April 24. Organised by the Primary Care Support Force with the Wells Park Health Project.

Jean Duerden • Gill Halksworth

Research Implementation
England

CHANGES IN PRACTICE

One of the most exciting aspects of the research (Stapleton et al 1998) has been the response of the English National Board to the report. They have worked extremely hard to implement the recommendations and have done so quite successfully, predominantly through the publication of two new booklets, launched at the ENB Conference on 20th May 1999.

The familiar yellow booklet *Supervision of Midwives – Advice and Guidance to Local Supervising Authorities and Supervisors of Midwives* has been radically updated. This update (ENB 1999a) introduces supervision within the New NHS and the part supervision of midwives will play in clinical governance. In introducing the recommendations from the research project, it refers to midwives being able to choose their own supervisor and it reminds supervisors of the need to guarantee confidentiality within the supervisory framework. There is an emphasis on empowerment in the supervisory relationship, encouraging an appeal mechanism against supervisory decisions and a deselection procedure for supervisors who fail to meet standards. Monitoring of each supervisor's performance is highlighted as a function of the LSA responsible officer.

Responding to the identified need to enhance the education of midwives on supervision is the Board's second publication *Supervision in Action* (ENB, 1999b), new booklet for midwives and student midwives to enable them to make more effective use of supervision. This booklet consolidates all the information on supervision given during training, so that midwives can make the best use of supervision and understand its purpose. The research (Stapleton et al, 1998) identified that this is particularly important at times of change in the structure or aims of supervision.

Supervision in Action pays attention to the supervision of midwives outside the clinical mainstream e.g. agency and bank midwives. The support role of the supervisor, especially after a clinical incident, is emphasised throughout, suggesting a no-blame culture. At the same time it reminds midwives of their own responsibilities and discourages dependence on supervisors. In this it responds to another of the recommendations in the report, to 'remove from the supervisory role any tasks which may encourage dependence and inhibit the empowerment of midwives'. The distinction between the role of the supervisor and the role of the manager, which confused many midwives interviewed for the project, is highlighted. Similarly, suspension from practice and suspension from duty is made clear.

Through these publications the Board have addressed the majority of the implications identified in the study:

1 The majority of midwives studied wished to choose their supervisor and the implementation of such choice would demonstrate a commitment to empowerment through supervision. There is also a need for balance between midwives' general desire for choice of supervisor and the supervisors' need for some choice in their case-load.

2 A guarantee of confidentiality is an essential foundation for trust in the supervisory relationship.

3 Where supervisors have strategies which enable midwives to experience supervision as empowering, those midwives feel that their practice is enhanced.

4 Supervisory decisions are empowering where they are made by consensus between supervisor and supervisee.

5 There is great potential for damage where supervision is experienced as intimidating. There is, therefore, a real need for mechanisms whereby allegations of bullying by a supervisor can be investigated as a matter of urgency. Supervisors who are found guilty of such behaviour should be deselected.

6 The creation of a mechanism of appeal against supervisory decisions would demonstrate commitment to fair and equitable practice and greatly enhance midwives' trust in the process of supervision.

7 Removal from the supervisory role of any tasks which may encourage dependence and inhibit the empowerment of midwives would enhance the effectiveness of supervision in the context of current practice.

8 Supervision and management roles could be clarified by ensuring that, in every case, the distinction between suspension from practice and suspension from duty is made clear to all concerned.

9 The establishment of mechanisms for the evaluation and monitoring of supervisory performance would be in keeping with the current aims and philosophy of supervision and clinical practice.

10 To ensure equity in the practice of supervision, it is essential that all midwives should be supervised and attention is paid to the supervision of midwives outside the clinical mainstream e.g. agency midwives.

11 To facilitate practice appropriate to women's needs, supervision should be appropriate to midwives' needs. Attention is particularly needed to ensure that supervision is appropriate to the needs of minority groups such as midwifery lecturers.

12 As the habits of blame and self-blame (which can give rise to scapegoating) are deeply ingrained in the culture of midwifery, supervision could model profound change by supporting a no-blame culture.

13 Historically, new tasks have been added to the work of supervisors without consideration for their total workload or the resulting conflicts within their role. It is, therefore, important that further responsibilities should be added to the work of supervisors only with great caution and with due attention to the effect of any addition on the overall workload.

Enhancing education on supervision for midwives

22 For midwives to make more effective use of supervision, they need a higher level of knowledge of supervision at qualification.

23 Education is required for qualified midwives so that they can make the best use of supervision and understand its purpose. This is particularly important at times of change in the structure or aims of supervision.

24 As ENB publications have been so successful in the education of supervisors, an ENB publication aimed at midwives and students would do much to meet the educational needs outlined.

The section of implications for supervisors of midwives (14-21) will no doubt be considered carefully when the open learning programme for the preparation of supervisors of midwives is next revised. Considering how closely the recommendations were followed in the new publications described above, there can be no doubt that similar scrutiny will be given to the research in such a revision and the recommendations included within the new publication.

Research implementation in Wales

During the actual research study in Wales it was clear that changes were being made in terms of the practice and role of the supervisor. To date, these changes are still occurring.

Ratio

There is a clear move to reducing the ratio of supervisors to midwives with an average of 1:17 being reported for the Principality. However, there is still a variety of practices with some areas evidently having a larger case-load and others endeavouring to move to a much smaller one. Indeed, one area is moving towards implementing a 1:10 ratio.

Appointment

The process of appointing supervisors is radically changing. In some areas peer elections are taking place, and the concept of applying and being interviewed for the post is becoming common practice. Many more clinicians are being appointed, the majority being G grade or above, although there have been appointments made at F grade.

Choice

Many units are moving towards midwives being able to choose their own supervisor or at least being given the option to choose three from those available, with whom they could relate and whom they would be willing to adopt as their supervisor.

Deselection

There is a move to address the problem of deselection of supervisors, with the consideration being on the individual midwife's evaluation as well as supervisor colleagues' opinions.

Separating the role

There has been a move by some supervisors to separate the different roles of supervision, namely supporter and investigator. Therefore, a supervisor would enact the roles of supporter, counsellor, friend and challenger to her/his own individual case-load. If an investigation was necessary for one of the midwives in her/his case-load, another supervisor would undertake the official investigation. The named supervisor would then be there to support the midwife throughout the investigation, being separate to the inquiry.

Role

There is a clear move towards the role being more a supportive and yet challenging one, rather than a reactive role. Education appears to be high on the agenda for many supervisors, whether it is through update programmes or formal continuing education courses. Risk management is also high on the agenda for many. Supervisors would appear to be becoming more politically aware and utilising their role as a supervisor to advance practice for the benefit of both the midwives and the women utilising the services.

The sand was clearly shifting during the research project itself and this shift has continued further. Supervision is no longer the total remit of managers, there is a clear move to the appointment of clinicians to the role, the ratio is being reduced and the role is fundamentally changing. Midwives would appear to be viewing supervision more positively than previously indicated. However, these are only observations, information gleaned and comments forwarded, following the completion of the original research project.

References

ENB. (1999a). *Advice and Guidance to Local Supervising Authorities and Supervisors of Midwives*. London: ENB.

ENB. (1999b). *Supervision in Action*. London: ENB.

Stapleton, H., Duerden, J., Kirkham, M. (1998). *Evaluation of the Impact of the Supervision of Midwives on Professional Practice and The Quality of Midwifery Care*. London: ENB.

Jean Duerden

The New LSA Arrangements
in Practice

CHANGES IN PRACTICE

This chapter will consider the new LSA arrangements in practice in England. At the end of the chapter the arrangements in the rest of the UK will be detailed for comparison.

The local supervising authority (LSA) is the body responsible by statute, for the general supervision of all midwives practising within its boundaries (ENB, 1999). Much has been written about the history of the supervision of midwives, not least by the editor of this book, and the role of the LSA responsible officer has been well described, especially from the perspective of the routine inspection of midwives which included inspection of her living arrangements and personal life (Heagerty, 1996). The profession of the person holding the position of the LSA responsible officer has changed over the years from the medical officer of health, over the first seventy years of supervision of midwives, followed by the regional health authority nurse for subsequent years until 1996 when all LSA officers' posts were taken by midwives.

Many of the tasks of responsible officers remain the same today as they did earlier this century, such as the receipt of notifications of intention to practise, the appointment of supervisors of midwives, determining whether to suspend a midwife from practice and investigating cases of alleged misconduct. The inspection of living arrangements and the personal lives of midwives are, happily, no longer the responsibilities of either LSA responsible officers or supervisors of midwives, as they were in the times that Heagerty described. Many new tasks, however, have been added to the role and there has been a different approach to carrying out the LSA role since each of the health authorities in England was designated as a local supervising authority by the Nurses, Midwives and Health Visitors Act 1997, Section 15 (1). This now means that the LSAs are accountable to the NHSE regional offices for exercising their statutory functions (ENB, 1999) and close liaison with the regional directors of nursing is maintained by officers.

In April 1996 there were 100 LSAs; there had been only eight regional LSAs prior to the Health Authorities Act 1995. The impracticality of having 100 LSA responsible officers meant that the health authorities grouped into consortia, with a responsible midwifery officer appointed to carry out the LSA function for each consortium. Each LSA is responsible for ensuring that statutory supervision of all midwives is exercised to a satisfactory standard within its geographical boundary.

The responsible officers appointed to each consortium were, and still are, all practising midwives professionally experienced in statutory supervision. The UKCC *Code of Practice*, when published in 1994, recommended that the designated responsible officer should be a midwife, emphasising the relationship between such a midwife and the local director of nursing/midwifery (UKCC, 1994 and 1998). Despite the recommendation being published in 1994, it was not until the new LSAs were formed in 1996 that a midwife held the LSA responsible officer role in every LSA. As midwives, the officers are able to provide a focus for issues relating to midwifery practice within each consortium boundary. As they are employed by each health authority, they are also able to contribute to the wider NHS agenda by supporting public health and inter-professional activities.

The role carries no management responsibility to trusts, neither does it represent the interests of the commissioners of maternity services. This unique position keeps the focus on midwifery practice, regardless of any budgetary restraints which might be imposed by trusts, and has an important influence on the quality of the local midwifery services. The most important aspect of the role is the regular contact with all supervisors of midwives.

To provide a national framework, the responsible midwifery officers have formed a national network of LSA officers, the LSA Midwifery Officers Forum. This forum provides a national picture of midwifery practice with information on contemporary issues and the wider NHS agenda. Through the Forum, the responsible officers are able to contribute informed advice on issues such as structures for local maternity services, manpower planning, student midwife numbers, post-registration education opportunities and many other issues, especially those referring to midwifery practice.

In addition to the national Forum meetings, the LSA officers meet collectively twice a year at the ENB with the director of midwifery education and practice, the assistant director of midwifery supervision and practice and the Board midwifery officers. Officers also meet twice yearly at the UKCC when the LSA officers and link supervisors from the other UK countries attend. There is also contact with the midwifery officer at the Department of Health. The support from the professional bodies for the LSA role cannot be overestimated.

Regular contact is made by the LSA officers with the health authority LSA representatives. Some representatives meet with their LSA officer as a consortium group, whilst other officers travel round their respective health authorities to meet with their executive officers who support the LSA function.

At the end of each year a local annual report is prepared by the responsible officers to outline the supervisory activities over the past year and report on audit outcomes and emerging trends affecting maternity services. This comprehensive report is communicated to all supervisors of midwives, the health authority, the NHSE regional office and the ENB. The report details how the statutory role of the LSA has been carried out. There is still a considerable amount of confusion about the role, even by the health authorities, despite the fact that they are now local supervising authorities. The report details how it has been possible to ensure that statutory supervision of midwives and midwifery practice is exercised to a satisfactory standard in order to secure appropriate midwifery care for every mother (ENB, 1999).

As clinical governance is high on every chief executive's agenda, there has been an increased interest in supervision. Each year the LSA officer makes a supervisory audit visit to each of the maternity units within the consortium to audit standards for supervision and midwifery practice. During these visits it has been possible to talk to chief executives about how the statutory function of supervision fulfils an important quality assurance remit, and how clinical effectiveness has been achieved in the maternity service.

There are many prescribed functions of the LSA to be discharged by the responsible midwifery officer and they are all listed in various texts, but probably most succinctly in the ENB (1999) publication *Advice and Guidance for Local Supervising Authorities and Supervisors* which has recently been updated.

Selection and appointment of supervisors

The appointment of appropriate numbers of supervisors of midwives is the first listed function and the word 'appropriate' is interpreted differently in each consortium. In Yorkshire, for example, a case-load of 15 midwives per supervisor is considered appropriate and that is the target across the county, although it has not yet been achieved in all trusts as staff retire, change roles or move hospitals. In the latter case, there would be a period of at least six months orientation to the new unit before an appointment as supervisor in that trust would be made.

The updated *Advice and Guidance* states that the LSA should produce 'guidelines for the process of nomination of prospective supervisors which will ensure that midwives are involved in the decision making process' (ENB 1999) and that 'guidelines for selection and appointment of prospective supervisors of midwives will demonstrate a process of equity'.

The nomination process is different within each consortium, and to a certain extent within each trust, although the West Midlands have an election process which is used across the consortium. Some supervisors warm to this idea, whilst others will not entertain it. At one trust in Yorkshire, elections were held recently and very successful nominations were made to the extent that the interview panel commented that they were the best candidates seen in a long time. They were not necessarily the supervisors' choice, but they certainly were the midwives' choice and their potential was clearly evident. The Board ask that the process should facilitate self- and peer-selection and recommend that a professional portfolio should be submitted as evidence of professional development.

The selection process at interview is equally important. The preparation course has shifted up an academic gear, and is now offered at Masters level in two universities as well as at levels two and three. No one wants to set a midwife up to fail, so it is crucial that the nominated midwife is capable of undertaking the course successfully. It still carries a fairly high failure rate. One of the common causes of failure is when a midwife fails to differentiate between supervision and management. It is, therefore, important that they can demonstrate ongoing professional development at a minimum of diploma level.

Each LSA has its own methods of selection, but the majority will include an interview by a panel which includes the LSA officer. The LSA officers use a common person specification for supervisors. Applicants must: have a minimum of three years' experience as a practising midwife of which at least one year has been in the period of two years immediately preceding the appointment (UKCC, 1998); have evidence of recent professional development at a minimum of diploma level; demonstrate the use of evidence to inform clinical practice; display leadership skills; have evidence of effective time management and display negotiation skills. Personal qualities must include: evidence of effective communication skills; good interpersonal skills; evidence of support from midwives; professionally credibility with midwives and the ability to maintain confidentiality of information. The desirable attributes are: having undertaken the ENB Course 997 'Teaching in Clinical Practice' or equivalent; a diploma or degree in midwifery studies; experience in all aspects of midwifery practice and an awareness of risk management issues.

The appointment process can be long after the initial nomination and selection as the preparation course and assessment can take up to nine months to complete, depending upon which centre the course is held at, and the Masters programme is, of course, even longer. Successful completion of the preparation course does not guarantee appointment. There have been occasions when midwives have proved during the preparation course that, for one reason or another, they are not ready to be appointed as supervisors. The appointment is then delayed until such time as both the prospective supervisor and the LSA officer feel comfortable about the appointment.

Once appointed, the new supervisors need their own support as well as providing it to the midwives on their case-load. The LSA officers ensure that these new supervisors have access to a support mechanism at all times. One model is to have quarterly meetings with the new supervisors in the first year of their appointment. This takes the form of a debriefing meeting where experiences are shared in a confidential arena, and the supervisors feel comfortable in the knowledge that they are not alone in feeling vulnerable or inept as they struggle with their new roles.

The Board also recommends a period of not less than six months' preceptorship. This preceptorship is crucial and can go wrong if the new supervisors themselves are not able to choose their own preceptor. In some units it is always the contact supervisor who feels obliged to take on the role and one can end up with the same situation as was identified in the research when student supervisors were provided with mentors from the 'old school' who had not undertaken the updated training.

Deselection of supervisors
The research (Stapleton et al, 1998) showed that midwives felt there was no recourse if a supervisor was not performing to the desired standard,

although it was not unknown for supervisors to be deselected in particular circumstances. The ENB now advise that a policy for the selection and deselection of supervisors is established by the LSA (ENB 1999), and that deselection should occur when the standard of supervision falls below that which is deemed acceptable by the LSA, or there is evidence of consistent failure by the supervisor as deemed by the annual audit. The final reason given for deselection in the new advice and guidance is again in response to the research: 'following investigation of complaints by midwives which have been substantiated'.

Number of supervisors of midwives

The UKCC currently recommend a ratio of not more than one supervisor per 40 midwives in the *Midwives Rules and Code of Practice* (para. 33, UKCC 1998). They say that this ratio 'allows both effective supervision and adequate support for midwives'. As supervision is, for most supervisors, part of a substantive midwifery post, the amount of time available to individual midwives with such a case-load is likely to be very small. The LSA officers in England are keen to reduce this ratio substantially and many have been successful – it has been reduced to 1:8 in one part of the Trent Region and is certainly in the low twenties in most areas.

Providing a framework of support

This function is open to various interpretations. Each LSA has its own guidelines for the supervision of midwives which are developed in various ways. Working groups of supervisors generally contribute to these guidelines which all have a local essence, and aim to promote the role of the supervisor in providing professional leadership, the empowerment of midwives, evidence-based practice, risk management, clinical audit and quality assurance (ENB, 1999). Acting on the research (Stapleton et al, 1998) the LSA endeavours to ensure that the guidelines produced ensure optimal participation of midwives and confidentiality within the supervisory relationship.

The standards for supervision, in addition to those provided by the ENB, are also locally prescribed so that they can be audited annually by the LSA officer during her supervisory audit visit. The standards can be expected to include equity, efficiency, effectiveness, accessibility and local acceptability (ENB, 1999). As the purpose of the supervisory audit visit is to evaluate the effectiveness of supervision of midwives and the practice of midwives, it is important that the standards prove to be a suitable benchmark for audit.

The framework is essentially one of communication and support for supervisors. Some of the consortia are so large that full meetings with all the supervisors are impractical. Supervisors have to travel long distances across large geographical areas for such meetings, which increases the length of time away from the workplace, and when all supervisors are released from work for such events, staffing within the maternity unit can be much reduced. Similarly, finding accommodation for a meeting of over 100 supervisors can generate its own difficulties. Emphasis is, therefore, given to local opportunities for meetings with other supervisors with a small delegation from each trust attending the full meetings. Regardless of the size of the meeting, opportunities are given for supervisors of midwives to debate professional issues and to gain information. Inevitably, it is at the smaller meetings where networking and peer support opportunities are at their optimum. The meetings may take the format of seminars, conferences or workshops.

In addition to the formal meetings, the LSA officer is available to support supervisors who should all know how to contact their responsible officer. This access is similarly available to midwives. In the past, it was unusual for a supervisor to contact the LSA unless she was referring a midwife for suspension. Happily, this is no longer the case and supervisors frequently contact the LSA for help and advice with practice problems.

Quality

It is common to include recommendations from national reports in supervisory audit visits, such as the Confidential Enquiry into Stillbirths and Deaths in Infancy (CESDI) and the Confidential Enquiry into Maternal Deaths (CEIMD). These regular reports provide excellent benchmarks for practice and implementation of recommendations can be audited.

Statistical information is also collected from each unit at the end of the year and a consortium profile of delivery rates, staffing levels, intervention rates, facilities etc. can be produced. As each LSA officer collates this information the national profile can similarly be monitored through the forum. The 12 officers in England are a frequently used resource for information which can quickly and efficiently be collated, often at one meeting. Each officer is well aware of maternity services in each of the trusts within her local consortium and a quick 'round robin' will often provide the information required.

One of the targets of LSA officers has been to ensure that supervision of midwives is included in all service level agreements with commissioners of maternity services. This has not been an easy task as it has not been an automatic inclusion when such agreements are drawn up, and because of the differing values placed on supervision. As many LSA officers are now in a position to provide advice and guidance on commissioning of maternity services at local level, the inclusion of supervision is now more acceptable.

Advisory role

Each LSA officer is employed by several health authorities in England, with each health authority contributing to part of the salary and overheads associated with the LSA responsible officer role. As such employees, the officers are also midwifery advisers to the health authorities. They can advise on preparing specifications for maternity services, on strategies for midwifery education and on UKCC, ENB and DoH national guidance and policy. As primary care groups have been formed, many LSA officers have been involved in providing midwifery advice to PCG chief executives and/or nurse board members, or at least identifying themselves as a resource.

Many LSA responsible officers sit on maternity service liaison committees, especially where these are combined meetings within each LSA. Here, again, the officer has an advisory role both to the health authority and to the represented trusts.

Notifications of intention to practise

Probably one of the most time-consuming roles is the receiving of notifications of intention to practise. As midwives are notoriously bad at filling in forms the amount of correction required, even after passing through the hands of their own supervisors, is phenomenal and very time-consuming. Each officer has to check thousands of these forms every year and the same mistakes are made time and again. Unsigned forms, the use of blue pen and correction fluid, and little notes scribbled to the UKCC on some part of the form are all regular anomalies, as are ticks instead of crosses, omissions and crossings out. From these forms, the local LSA database is compiled so that each LSA has ready information about all midwives practising in the consortium. This is updated monthly with the new notifications and changes of names and addresses. Secretarial support varies around the country and it is not unknown for officers to have to compile their own database.

Through the receipt of the notifications, another statutory duty is fulfilled: to ensure that each midwife meets the statutory requirements for practice. Again, it is surprising how many notifications are received that show that a midwife has not undertaken any statutory update for seven years or more. Sometimes this is a clerical error, but there are midwives who continue to be unaware of their statutory responsibility for professional update and the nannying referred to in the research (Stapleton et al, 1998) becomes a necessity.

Providing education and training for supervisors

The LSA midwifery officer is responsible for ensuring that prospective supervisors have access to a preparation course and to continuing education thereafter, in accordance with Rule 44 (UKCC, 1998). Within each consortium, there is a university which facilitates the preparation course and supports the ongoing education programme for supervisors. Many officers are honorary lecturers at those universities. Some consortia form an education consortium to offer the preparation course more frequently, e.g. the Northern, Yorkshire and Trent consortia are able to offer three courses a year in Newcastle, Leeds and Sheffield respectively, providing frequent access to courses with a common programme and assessment strategy.

The LSA officers nominate assessor supervisors to support student supervisors to ensure they are appropriately prepared for this role and able to carry it out in a competent and supportive manner, and to enable effective preparation of the nominated supervisor for her role. A mentorship preparation workshop prior to undertaking this role is also facilitated.

Continuing education is generally provided at a more local level. There once were residential refresher courses for supervisors of one week's duration until a change in the rules which required that supervisors undertook 15 hours of professional update in midwifery supervision every three years (Rule 44, *Midwives Rules*, UKCC 1998). Some three-day residential courses continue, but many LSAs now provide study days on supervisory topics once or twice a year, as well as other opportunities for update at local meetings, which may include speakers on specific, relevant topics.

Managing communications within supervisory systems

It is sometimes appropriate to describe the LSA officer as a glorified post box, as disseminating information from the statutory bodies is another of the statutory responsibilities. This information can be anything from the list of professionals removed from the register, from the UKCC, to hazard notices from the Department of Health. Working with health authorities also provides prompt receipt of health service circulars and those relevant to midwifery can be copied out to contact supervisors. Information gleaned at national meetings, such as those held at the ENB, the UKCC or the national Forum meetings, can also be distributed promptly through LSA briefings or similar newsletters.

Investigating cases of alleged misconduct

This is not, happily, a large part of the LSA role, in particular, determining whether to suspend a midwife from practice, in accordance with Rule 38 of the *Midwives Rules* (UKCC 1998). It is though, perhaps, the role for which LSA officers are most easily recognised, although in 1997 no midwives were removed from the register. When midwives are asked what they believe the role to be, they will frequently quote the suspension of midwives, and yet there are many officers who have never suspended a midwife from practice and hope never to do so. With proactive supervision, many of these cases can be avoided, and, where a midwife shows evidence of poor practice, appropriate supervisory intervention can pay dividends. The most important aspect, in the first instance, is recognition by the midwife of substandard practice. The natural reaction of most midwives is to be defensive in these circumstances, and the skills of a supervisor are paramount in handling the situation.

Where critical incidents have involved the substandard practice of a midwife, the supervisor undertaking the inquiry into the incident may contact the LSA for advice and guidance. It is rare that the advice would be to proceed with a report to recommend the suspension of the midwife from practice. The most common support offered, in these circumstances, is help with drafting the supervisory learning contract appropriate to the incident and personal learning needs of the individual midwife. Supervisors themselves often feel vulnerable during this period of investigation, particularly if the midwife herself is in complete denial and believes she is being victimised.

Where a midwife can be made aware of her lack of knowledge and skills, the most appropriate action is for a period of supervised practice with a learning contract drafted as in Case Study 3 in Chapter 9. With the support of her supervisor, a midwife can undertake a programme of learning and re-skilling and grow from the process, increasing her self-value and esteem, as well as that of her colleagues. Through this supervisory process, many midwives have learned from their mistakes and gone on to higher levels of education as a result of their exposure to new ideas and training. Some have become supervisors themselves or sought promotion along other avenues. This is a far superior approach to that of suspension and the persecution that that brings.

Responding again to the research (Stapleton et al, 1998), the ENB now recommends that the LSA establishes a mechanism for appeal against supervisory decisions to promote openness (ENB, 1999).

Despite this proactive approach, one cannot turn a blind eye to the fact that there are some midwives who cannot see the error of their ways and continue to present a risk to the public. Where care of women is severely compromised and other women are at risk from the particular practice of a midwife, then an LSA officer has no option but to suspend the midwife concerned from practice and refer her to the UKCC Professional Conduct Committee. Similarly, where the health of a midwife affects the care she gives to women, or if she is guilty of a criminal offence, referral must also be made either to the UKCC Health Committee or the Professional Conduct Committee.

In these situations, each LSA officer ensures that supervisors of midwives are able to demonstrate that investigations of alleged suboptimal care or professional misconduct have been carried out in an impartial and confidential manner. Outcomes of investigations are communicated to all the relevant bodies. The health authorities receive a report on cases of alleged misconduct where the midwife has been reported to the

Professional Conduct Committee of the UKCC and are notified of further developments until the case is concluded.

Maternal deaths

All maternal deaths are reported to the LSA officer. Each officer has prepared guidelines to be used in the event of a maternal death. The officers report maternal deaths to the Director of Public Health at the relevant health authority and to the Department of Health for the Confidential Enquiry into Maternal Deaths. This is a 'belt and braces' approach as there are other mechanisms in place for such reporting, but, as many had been missed and not reported to the Department, a request was made to the officers to take on this reporting role to avoid omissions and this has met with success.

Direct midwifery contribution to education

The duties of the LSA officer include ensuring that there are comprehensive education and training opportunities available to all midwives and supervisors of midwives, contributing to the development of midwifery education and, as appropriate, participating in the delivery of education programmes for supervisors and midwives (ENB, 1999). Several LSA officers are members of the education consortium within their consortia and are able to influence the provision of midwifery education. They also endeavour to have membership of relevant curriculum design teams and to participate in validation events as appropriate. Thus, midwifery is represented at a senior level on curriculum design teams both pre- and post-registration.

Return to midwifery practice

The LSA responsible officers provide career advice for midwives who are considering returning to midwifery practice. Their individual requirements are assessed in accordance with ENB guidance. The officers work with the relevant education consortia and universities to ensure that there is local provision of return to midwifery practice programmes. The demand for such courses varies across the country, as does the funding. As the shortage of midwives increases, encouragement for midwives considering return to midwifery practice is crucial, with easy access to appropriate courses and as much financial support as possible. When women's salaries contribute to mortgage payments, it is very difficult to encourage anyone to give up full time work to undertake a course of approximately three months which offers no salary, but is practice based. This situation is currently changing as the government has made new money available to support those returning to practice to reduce such financial loss.

Link supervisors

Not every LSA has link supervisors, but where they are appointed they are experienced supervisors of midwives and provide a valuable service by assisting the LSA in carrying out its statutory function. The title 'link' may be somewhat inappropriate now as it used to refer to the link between supervisors of midwives and the LSA. There is now direct communication with, and easy access to, all the LSA officers for every supervisor. The role, therefore, is much more as a deputy during absence and as a sounding board for the LSA officer in her isolated role. They help to make strategic decisions about supervision within their consortium and give expert advice and support.

Clinical governance

The three key aspects of setting, delivering and monitoring standards are described in *First Class Service* (DoH 1998, 1.16) as professional self-regulation, clinical governance and lifelong learning. None of these is new to midwives as they have all been integral to the supervision of midwives. LSA officers are, therefore, in a position to promote supervision as a tool for clinical governance as it empowers midwives to work within the full scope of their role, offering a framework for scrutiny of professional standard practice, through a non-confrontational, confidential, midwife led review of a midwife's level of knowledge, understanding and competence (ENB, 1999).

Supervisors are expected to promote and develop safe practice and ensure the dissemination of good, evidence-based practice and innovation. Since 1955, the supervision of midwives has ensured a statutory framework for continued professional development and compulsory refreshment of midwifery knowledge has led to a lifelong learning programme for midwives throughout their careers. The supervisory review provides the formal focus of support and reflection with a confidential review of professional development needs. Supervision, therefore, contributes to an effective framework of clinical governance which minimises risk and reduces patient complaints. Supervisors are now part of multi-disciplinary teams which collaborate to produce practice guidelines.

Through the National Institute for Clinical Excellence (NICE) established on 1st April 1999, clear national standards will be set, backed by consistent monitoring arrangements. The 12 LSA responsible midwifery officers, through their supervisory audit visits to each maternity unit, regularly monitor standards of practice against documented evidence such as that produced by the CESDI, CEIMD and the Royal College of Obstetricians *Effective Procedures in Maternity Care Suitable for Audit*. As other national yardsticks and standards are developed through national service frameworks and NICE, any pertaining to maternity services can continue to be monitored in this way. Where there are unacceptable variations in clinical midwifery practice, or care is inappropriate for women's needs, the LSA responsible midwifery officer, as an outside assessor, is in a position to recommend remedial action. Similarly, the LSA can contribute to the dissemination of information from NICE to ensure the implementation of the most effective care.

First Class Service (DoH 1998) describes a clinical governance framework (3.11) that will modernise and strengthen professional self-regulation and build on the principles of performance. Annual supervisory reviews assess midwifery practice and identify knowledge gaps. These are then addressed by facilitating appropriate professional development.

The clinical governance framework is also intended to strengthen existing systems for quality control, based on clinical standards, evidence-based practice and learning the lessons of poor performance. Through supervisory audit, all these aspects are met. The supervisors are able to identify good practice and share this through the supervisory network.

A further target of clinical governance is to assess and minimise the risk of untoward events. All untoward events involving midwives are recorded, investigated and monitored by supervisors. Development needs are identified and professional development programmes facilitated.

Another clinical governance initiative is to investigate problems as these arise and ensure lessons are learnt. Critical incident analysis, as described above, is a crucial part of the supervisor's role. The document calls for clinical governance to support health professionals in delivering quality care. One of the principal functions of supervision is to provide support for midwives.

The professional self-regulation of midwives is supported by the supervision of midwives. Matters of alleged professional misconduct are dealt with through the supervisory channel. The responsibility of LSA officers is to promote the role of the supervisor in risk management, clinical audit, quality assurance, education and training, evidence-based practice and professional leadership at every trust and health authority in each consortium. With its long-established function, statutory supervision of midwives is well prepared to make a substantial contribution to the clinical governance framework within maternity services.

The LSA responsible officer role in other UK countries

The above has been an impression of the LSA role in England. An LSA responsible officer from each of the other three UK countries was approached and asked to detail the differences in their role from the role described above.

LSA officer role in Scotland

In Scotland there are 15 LSAs, each health board being an LSA. The LSA responsible officer is not necessarily a midwife: in fact there is only one midwife holding such a role, and in all others the LSA representative is a nurse at health board level, either the director of nursing or quality. The midwife LSA responsible officer has one four-hour session per week allocated to undertake the role.

The LSA responsible officers produce biennial reports to the NBS which are passed on to all supervisors of midwives. The reports are developed from their annual audit of local standards and practice development reports from each hospital. Statistical information is collected and collated by the Information Service Division at the Scottish Office. The LSA officers receive the notifications of intention to practise from the supervisors, pass on communications from the UKCC and NBS to all supervisors, receive notifications of maternal deaths, and hold quarterly meetings with the supervisors within their LSA. Copies of the NBS professional officers' report of the three-yearly audit visit are submitted to the relevant LSA with action points. These are subsequently audited at the next LSA annual audit.

There are 16 link supervisors in Scotland and they perform much of the LSA function described earlier in this chapter, such as investigating matters of alleged professional misconduct and promoting the role of the supervisor in risk management, and provide more of the advisory role to the responsible officers. They are members of maternity services liaison committees and health gain commissioning teams and work very closely with the LSA representatives. They attend UKCC LSA responsible officers' meetings rather than the LSA officers. The link supervisors in Scotland have their own informal network.

There are annual seminars run by the National Board of Scotland (NBS) where relevant issues are debated. A current issue is the Scotland-wide standard for selection, appointment and deselection of supervisors of midwives.

The current ratio of supervisors to midwives is 1:30-35, but is as low as 1:20 in some areas. Link supervisors have responsibility for the supervision of midwives in anything from two city hospitals to six small maternity units in the Highlands and Islands.

Guidelines for supervision are provided by the NBS. Standards for supervision are UK-wide and, as the National Institute for Clinical Excellence (NICE) is established in England, the Scottish equivalent the Clinical Standards Board for Scotland has just appointed an LSA responsible officer to its board.

LSA officer role in Wales

In Wales the health authorities are currently designated as the local supervising authorities. As in Scotland, there is an LSA representative at each health authority and a practising midwife has been appointed to carry out the supervisory role, designated as the 'lead supervisor of midwives'; one area has two midwives sharing the responsibility due to the geographical difficulties in this area.

The current lead supervisors are also midwifery managers and undertake LSA work on a notional one or two days a week. The hours spent on LSA duties are reimbursed to the employing trust by the Health Authority. In real terms, the lead supervisors do LSA work 'as required', on a flexible basis. Maternity statistics are collated by the All Wales Midwifery Network Group. These are used within trusts, etc. for audit purposes.

There are varying numbers of trusts providing maternity services in each health authority and the title link supervisor is given to the contact supervisor in each trust who is usually the head of midwifery or the senior midwife. The lead supervisors in Wales are able to fulfil all the roles described in this chapter, although there is currently no policy for the deselection of a supervisor of midwives. Notifications of intention to practise are handled exactly as in England and Scotland. The current ratio of supervisors to midwives varies but averages about 1:20.

There are close working relationships in Wales between the lead supervisors, the Welsh National Board (WNB), and the Welsh Office Nursing Division, with regular meetings. The WNB is charged with the same responsibility as the ENB to provide advice and guidance on matters relating to the statutory supervision of midwives.

The lead supervisors recognised that the constitutional changes (which have resulted in the National Assembly for Wales) gave them an opportunity to raise the profile of midwifery supervision. One way of doing this was to develop Wales-wide midwifery supervision polices, guidelines and standards. This would also ensure a consistent approach to midwifery supervision, built on best practice. The lead supervisors have built on the existing health authority policies. The first part of this new collaborative policy will be presented to health authorities by July 1999, and subject to the agreement of the health authorities, will now be adopted. Further standards will be developed using the same collaborative model over the next year.

LSA officer role in Northern Ireland

There are currently four health boards in Northern Ireland and each is a local supervising authority. Uniquely in Northern Ireland, the health boards are health and personal social services boards (HPSS). At present, only one of these boards has a midwifery officer at board level. In all cases, the regional officer is a nurse, but the link supervisors, heads of midwifery from a trust in each health board area, provide advice to the LSA and endeavour to fulfil the functions described above. There are 13 maternity units, a number which has recently reduced and is likely to continue to reduce. There are from two to six maternity units per HPSS.

There is no allocated time for the link supervisor role and no financial recompense for work undertaken to the respective trust from the HPSS.

As a result, the link supervisors believe they are unable to carry out the role as fully as they wish, and certainly not to the extent of the LSA role in England.

The ratio of supervisors to midwives is just under 1:40, but can vary from 22 to more than 40. The link supervisors have an excellent network between the trusts. There is currently no real selection process for supervisors. Nomination is by heads of midwifery and there is no interview process. They do, however, have to successfully complete the preparation course for prospective supervisors of midwives and then meet with the link supervisor for a 'one to one' prior to appointment. A selection and deselection process is currently being drafted.

The link supervisors check the notifications of intention to practise and submit them to the HPSS where they are collated on to a database. Link supervisors investigate allegations of misconduct, but the regional LSA officer makes any referrals to the UKCC.

The LSA structure is likely to change in the future, following the publication of the government's proposals for the future of health and personal social services in Northern Ireland (DHSS 1999).

LSA officer role in Jersey

The LSA officer in Jersey covers the whole of the Jersey maternity service. There are no Department of Health requirements, but the officer chooses to follow their recommendations. Jersey is not part of the United Kingdom, but a British Isle and only UKCC registered midwives are employed. The supervisory structure is the same as in England and there is one LSA officer and four supervisors for the island. The officer works with the medical officer of health of Jersey States Health and Social Services Committee on professional issues and acts as midwifery adviser. The LSA officer is a civil servant, but is paid by the States Health as are all midwives, but the salary incorporates the LSA function. There is resource and support for supervision in Jersey. The LSA officer meets quarterly with the supervisors to deal with clinical concerns and practice and also meets with the South and West Region LSA group in England for sharing, education, networking and to avoid alienation. There is occasional contact with Guernsey which is part of the South and West LSA Consortium.

There is no statutory accountability to the UKCC and no legal requirement to notify intention to practise as a midwife. However, Jersey has notification of intention to practise forms, not UKCC forms and the LSA officer collects and collates these.

Review of the Nurses, Midwives and Health Visitors Act

At the time of writing this chapter, the ongoing role of the LSA responsible officer is unclear, even to the extent of whether or not there will continue to be such a role in the future. With the demise of the national boards, there will still be many statutory duties to be carried out and who will take responsibility for those duties is yet to be determined. The future of statutory supervision is also unclear at the present time, as the impact and implementation of clinical governance has to be evaluated before decisions about the future of supervision are made. LSA officers must continue to develop their role and prove the value of the supervision of midwives.

References

Department of Health. (1998). *A First Class Service*. London: HMSO.

DHSS. (1999). *Fit for the Future: A New Approach, The Government's Proposals for the Future of the Health and Personal Social Services in Northern Ireland*. Northern Ireland: DHSS.

ENB. (1999). *Advice and Guidance to Local Supervising Authorities and Supervisors of Midwives*. London: ENB.

Heagerty, B.V. (1996). 'Reassessing the guilty: The Midwives Act and the control of English midwives in the early 20th century'. In: Kirkham, M. *Supervision of Midwives*. Hale: Books for Midwives Press.

Stapleton, H., Duerden, J., Kirkham, M. (1998). *Evaluation of the Impact of the Supervision of Midwives on Professional Practice and The Quality of Midwifery Care*. London: ENB.

UKCC. (1998). *Midwives Rules and Code of Practice*. London: UKCC.

Olive Jones

Supervision in a Midwife Managed Birth Centre

CHANGES IN PRACTICE

When executed effectively, supervision develops professional leadership which creates a practice environment to support innovation and where midwives develop new roles to practise autonomously and contribute to cost effective ways of achieving woman centred care. (ENB 1996)

This chapter will explore the place of the dynamic process of midwifery supervision in introducing a new maternity service and building a consensual approach to care, and will examine how midwifery supervision has been a key element in developing loyalty to quality care and changing attitudes to practice. Key areas which will be addressed are the development and implementation of evidence-based guidelines, learning in the workplace, group-guided reflection on practice and critical incident analysis. To illustrate particular points, use has been made of the reflective writing of midwives working in the birth centre.

This project preceded the present government's plans for a 'New NHS' (DoH 1997a); however, it fits well with the concept of different trusts and different professions working in partnership, in terms of meeting the needs of clients as the competitive element which arose from internal marketing is removed.

Background

There are a number of birth centres scattered around the country. Usually they are to be found in rural areas several miles from hospital services. As part of rationalisation of services, many are under threat of closure. Edgware birth centre is unusual in that it is a new venture in this climate and is situated in an urban area in close proximity to several hospital obstetric units. It is unique in that three trusts, Wellhouse which is the host trust, Northwick Park and St Mark's and Royal Free, collaborate in providing a service to local women on a site managed by a fourth trust, Barnet Healthcare. Midwifery supervision crosses boundaries involving three districts and two local supervising authorities (LSAs). Supervisors of midwives from these districts and the responsible officers of the two LSAs contributed to the process of setting up the birth centre.

The announcement in 1996 of a change in status of Edgware General from acute to community hospital met with public dismay. The local maternity services liaison committee, encouraged by acceptance at government level (DoH 1992, DoH 1993) of midwifery managed units, saw an opportunity to improve choice for women and became a major driving force of the birth centre initiative. A survey of local women was commissioned which suggested that 61.6 per cent of those suitable would consider using a birth centre geographically separated from an acute hospital (Manero, 1997). An expert advisory panel comprised of nominated representatives from appropriate professional colleges heard evidence from key professionals and lay organisations. The proposal for the birth centre was accepted and central funding of a demonstrator project was granted for two years with a condition that the project would be independently evaluated.

Invitations to midwives employed by the host trust to participate in the project met with a disappointing response. There was a political agenda associated with the closure of Edgware General Hospital which became a general election issue. Consequently there was an element of opportunism in grasping a moment which may not have presented again. With a tight time-frame for planning and implementing change, staff had not had time to accept an ending to what they had known in Edgware; this may have accounted for their reluctance to accept a new beginning (Tichy and Ulrich, 1984). The response to national advertising was overwhelming. An enthusiastic team of midwives, drawn from existing resources and new appointments, was recruited to the project.

There is a small core team of midwives and midwifery assistants who provide 24-hour cover in the birth centre. This team is encouraged to be self-managing within predetermined boundaries. One midwife co-ordinates the activities of the birth centre staff and 'visiting midwives' from the three participating trusts who access the birth centre to care for women. The other midwives have defined responsibilities within their role; one is a supervisor of midwives. This non-hierarchical structure works well and staff particularly appreciate being able to decide their working pattern so as to be as family-friendly as possible whilst maximising continuity of carer for women. Midwives are accountable to a senior midwifery manager, based in the consultant unit of the host trust, from whom they can seek advice and who ensures that information is shared with them and that they do not become marginalised through their geographical separation from the main line service.

A guiding principle is that nothing will be undertaken in the birth centre unless it could be done with confidence in the woman's own home. There are no medical staff on site. In the event of complications arising the woman is transferred by ambulance with paramedic support to one of the three participating consultant units. The birth centre does not vie with birth at home or in a consultant unit; emphasis is very much on extending choice for women by working in partnership with midwifery and medical colleagues in both primary and secondary care settings.

Resistance

Change releases negative and positive forces; it would be misleading to suggest that there was no resistance to the birth centre proposal. Whilst there has been overwhelming support, sometimes from unexpected quarters, there has also been resistance from professionals. An isolated, midwife managed service does not conform to the perceived norm, leading to uncertainty about its function. Some general practitioners and midwives voiced concern and demonstrated resistance, not so much to the concept of a midwife managed birth centre but to it being geographically separated from consultant services. 'It is unsafe' has been the most common cry. The concept of safety is complex; a measure of clinical outcomes is often used as a parameter and appropriate research findings (Campbell and Macfarlane 1994, Hundley et al 1994, Baird et al 1996) were considered by the expert advisory panel in reaching a decision to approve the proposal for the centre.

General practitioners and midwives are very effective 'gatekeepers' to health services and can subtly assume control of the woman's childbirth experience by withholding information. It was apparent that not all midwives gave women information about the birth centre. This has been overcome by giving women an information leaflet before their booking appointment. It sets out all options available and asks the woman to identify those she wishes to discuss with her midwife. On more than one occasion general practitioners have attempted to obstruct women who want to give birth in the centre and sought to cancel arrangements made (Walker, 1998). Regardless of women meeting strict acceptance criteria, the physical safety of mother and baby is deemed to be at risk, a view expressed without supporting evidence. Psychological factors appear to be ignored. A couple who discovered the birth centre half way through

Figure 7.1: A Framework for Midwifery Supervision

Group reflection
guidelines tested in practice.

Evidence-based guidelines are developed
in a collaborative framework.

By promoting individual self-esteem and
professional development, midwives can
be empowered to extend their boundaries
of knowledge and practice.

Women and their families are at the
centre of care and full participants
in decision making.

All members of staff are valued. Excellence
in practice is the aim.

Midwifery supervision is the core
of a dynamic process.

their pregnancy argued cogently against the ethics of a claim to offer informed choice while control over decision making is maintained by limiting options. They stated they felt empowered when told by their doctor that they could choose where the baby would be born; however, as soon as they mentioned home they were told this was not an option for them in a first pregnancy. The birth centre was not offered as a choice. Immediately they felt disempowered. They were critical of attempts to seduce them to conform in the absence of research-based information and suggested such a patriarchal approach was insulting to them.

A small number of general practitioners were concerned that they would be vicariously responsible if their patients experienced an unfavourable outcome of care in the birth centre. The General Medical Services Committee published guidance on intrapartum care for general practitioners (1996) in which it stated that general practitioners should give impartial evidence-based advice to enable women to make an informed choice about their care even if their choice is contrary to the personal view of the doctor. It further makes explicit that the doctor can choose whether or not to contract with the woman to provide intrapartum care and that there is no obligation to do so when a contract for antenatal care is made.

It has been important for the supervisor of midwives to initiate debate to dispel myths and challenge beliefs which have no foundation in research. There was consensus that a desired outcome cannot be guaranteed wherever birth takes place; this was an important principle in taking the debate forward. The most appropriate analogy is drawn with home birth. The confidential enquiry into home birth conducted in 1994 (Chamberlain et al, 1997) concluded that women who fall into a low risk category should be allowed to give birth at home although it was acknowledged that some would develop complications and require transfer to a consultant unit. Strict acceptance criteria are in place for the centre and, unlike home birth, women cannot insist on delivery in a birth centre (Dimond and Walters, 1997). Thus it is not appropriate to make comparisons with unplanned home birth which was associated with unfavourable outcomes in the enquiry. As with the home birth debate, that of the birth centre is likely to run and run.

Philosophy

The voice of the supervisor of midwives was at the core of the development process, acting as a link, crossing organisational and institutional boundaries. *Changing Childbirth* (DoH, 1993) was a trigger to indicate much needed change in the way maternity services were provided. The nature of a demonstrator project and the appointment of a supervisor of midwives as project leader offered an opportunity for midwifery supervision to activate the trigger and come to the fore in facilitating the empowerment of midwives as autonomous practitioners in a practice setting, geographically separated from an acute hospital site.

Once the core team was identified, they and community based midwives from the three participating trusts were invited to meet with the project leader. Midwives were presented with the vision to which they had committed themselves when joining the project and each one was asked to write what she considered the philosophy of the birth centre should be. A mission statement was created entirely based on this, thus fostering from the outset the fact that everyone has something of value to offer to fundamental organisation and drawing together the personal aspirations of all those involved. The many and varied backgrounds from which midwives came could have driven a wedge between them. It was important that a supervisory thread be woven into the very fabric of this new venture from the beginning. It is believed that this was crucial to enable a cohesiveness to develop and promote the notion of three trusts building a consensual approach to care.

Edgware Birth Centre opened in September 1997. The centre, a 'stand alone' facility, geographically isolated from consultant obstetric services by 6 to 8 miles, midwife managed with no medical input, extends choice for women who meet the acceptance criteria and actively choose a birth without intervention in a home from home setting. The adopted philosophy is one of empowerment of women and carers and reflects the ideals of *Changing Childbirth* (DoH, 1993) in terms of choice, continuity and control for women. In practice, this has evolved into a concept of family centred care as partners, children and grandparents intimately share in this major life event. Women and families are at the forefront of care; midwives seek to facilitate informed choice and foster a non-intrusive, non-interventionist approach to birth. The aim is that through evidence-based practice, spontaneous birth is supported with confidence and competence with women feeling safe, confident and totally involved in all aspects of their care regardless of background, culture or religious belief.

In this context, the aim of supervision was for midwives to be empowered as autonomous practitioners in providing care which women want. A pragmatic approach to supervision was agreed between the two LSA responsible officers and supervisors of the three trusts. As well as each midwife having a named supervisor in her employing trust, there would be a named supervisor for the birth centre to whom midwives, students, midwifery assistants and others would have access. This supervisor would liaise with the named supervisors of midwives when indicated. A philosophical framework for supervision evolved (see Figure 7.1). The focus was on collaborative working between trusts, underpinned by a belief that by promoting individual self-esteem and professional development, midwives can be empowered to extend their boundaries of knowledge and practice to the benefit of women and their families and, in turn, empowering them by helping them to achieve the childbirth experience to which they aspire.

Determining boundaries of expertise

It was agreed that guidelines were necessary to assist midwives as lead professionals in delivering woman centred care in an isolated practice setting. Guidelines can be found in almost any maternity unit although the notion of evidence-based guidelines is relatively new to midwifery. Shennan (in Kirkham, 1996) reported examples of midwives being disabled by rigid policies which became a master rather than a tool for practice. Similarly, some midwives who joined the birth centre project cited experiences of being previously constrained in practice and unable to meet the wishes of women because of prescriptive policies which were not underpinned by research. Such rigid policies raise an issue of power; they allow the carer to assume control of childbirth, legitimising authority over women. There is the potential for midwives to act by rote without thinking about what they are doing or why. Midwives were anxious to avoid such a situation in the birth centre.

It was considered important that midwives should be able to decide what guidelines they would use and be actively involved in the development and implementation of these guidelines. To enable them in this activity they needed to understand the theory underpinning the design and use of guidelines. Whilst they were encouraged to undertake the work themselves, the supervisor was available to give advice on the process.

Garcia and Garforth (1991) report that midwives need a structure in which to work for efficient functioning and that midwives value involvement in policy making. They stress the need to apply routines flexibly to meet the needs of women and carers. Kirkham (1996a) is critical of protocols which are not research-based and often developed in response to disasters, which limit the scope for professional decision making and do not support individualised care for women.

Price and Price (1997) suggest that midwives make intuitive decisions often unaware of their experiential knowledge, the theory and research upon which they draw when making decisions. That to which women aspire in their birth experience and respect for their values is also likely to be a factor in professional decision making. Evidence-based guidelines present an opportunity to implement research findings in practice and provide a framework for midwives to make sound clinical decisions. Making an evidence-based decision is arguably about achieving a desired outcome. Guidelines and systematic review of practice provide a basis for a clinical judgement process which is transparent; this is particularly important when complications arise and the midwife must account for her actions.

Guidelines for managing emergency situations are essential (DoH 1996, DoH 1997, Lewis and Dodds 1997), especially in an isolated practice setting without immediate recourse to medical aid where it is imperative that midwives can act swiftly and effectively to preserve the life and well-being of mothers and babies. The fourth CESDI report (DoH, 1997b), when identifying suboptimal care, was critical of carers ignoring established guidelines. Thus guidelines are integral to risk management.

The roots of risk management strategies adopted by trusts lie in insurance primarily to reduce the incidence of compensation claims (Dineen, 1997). Dineen reports a lower incidence of disciplinary action when guidelines are used. Obstetric litigation costs run into millions of pounds, money which could better be spent on clinical care in a financially constrained health service. Midwifery supervision, with its primary function of protecting the public from unsafe practice, cannot be separated from risk management and the supervisor has an important role in developing and implementing guidelines for practice.

The legal aspects of guidelines are worthy of examination. Litigious action is not the sole province of medical practice. Flint (1997) describes the trauma experienced by midwives, regardless of the outcome, against whom action is taken. Midwives are accountable to women, the United Kingdom Central Council and employers who assume vicarious liability, for acts of commission and omission in practice. Guidelines provide a standard for courts and as they increase in use are likely to be referred to in legal action although they would need to be supported by expert witnesses as reflecting contemporary practice (Hurwitz, 1995). It is unlikely they would be viewed as replacing clinical judgement which must satisfy the 'Bolam' test

(1957) but nevertheless those who write guidelines are accountable as well as users and it is a point of good practice to document the process. Hurwitz reports that in the United States of America, developers of faulty guidelines could be held liable if patients suffer harm as a result of clinicians adhering to them. Newdick (1997) argues this would be unlikely in the UK where clinicians would be expected to know if a guideline is applicable or not. Midwives have a responsibility to be clinically up to date and to work within employers' guidelines which should enable the best care for mothers and babies (UKCC 1993, 1994). It follows that if guidelines are not complied with for some reason, for example, because they conflict with the wishes of a woman, record keeping is of the highest significance so that the rationale for decision making is transparent, particularly if court action ensues. Record keeping was a particular area where midwives identified they wanted support from supervisors in order for their practice to stand up to scrutiny.

Purchasers and providers of care and supervisors of midwives are all concerned with quality of services, although their focus may differ. Valid and reliable evidence-based guidelines can be an important component in a strategy to enhance care for women and their families. Validity and reliability are determined by the evidence base and the same outcome being achieved by each user. There may also be cost savings if changes in practice result in improved outcomes (Grimshaw et al, 1995). Humphris and Littlejohns (1996) list several components necessary to the successful implementation of guidelines. These include a structured process, identified philosophy, open and collaborative dialogue, and professionals motivated to change practice.

At the birth centre, much time was saved by seeking permission to use guidelines for midwife led care of normal labour developed and tested in another trust (Leicester Royal Infirmary, 1997). To complement these, midwives with an interest in key areas were identified to take the lead (lead midwife) in developing guidelines for use in emergency situations.

Following a selected literature review, critical appraisal of relevant research was undertaken. Particular attention was paid to methodology to grade the research and the environment of each study to assess whether it was applicable to transfer research findings to practice in a birth centre. Utilisation of the Cochrane database was helpful at this point. A synthesis of research knowledge provided an opportunity for learning and professional development. The lead midwife collated research evidence and designed the guidelines for emergency situations, circulating draft copies to key stakeholders for comments. Advice was sought from appropriate specialists: obstetricians, paediatricians, anaesthetists, the trust senior nurse for resuscitation who took the lead in developing guidelines for that purpose, the senior neonatal nurse and London Ambulance Service. Thus action to be taken to treat and transfer in the event of complications arising would be acceptable to the receiving consultant unit. Consultant medical staff readily collaborated with midwives in developing guidelines and offered valuable suggestions. A culture of mutual respect was fostered.

Guidelines should be written in unambiguous language making explicit mandatory and non-mandatory actions; given the same circumstances each professional should interpret them in the same way (Grimshaw and Russell, 1993). Current thinking on the topic through referenced selected literature should be included and linked to the different approaches to management of care described, so that the practitioner may select an appropriate option. Guidelines should inform, rather than restrict, clinical practice (Newdick, 1996); assist, not replace, clinical judgement (West and Newton, 1997). For normal situations they need to be flexible enough to allow deductive reasoning and to meet the needs of midwives and individual women or there is a risk that care may become depersonalised. Management of emergencies in childbirth requires more rigid guidance to ensure a consistent approach to care. A choice of options conveys accountability and the rationale for decisions made should be reflected in record keeping. A template for writing up notes was included as an appendix to each guideline related to the management of emergency situations in order to ensure a uniform record in all circumstances. When the final draft stage was reached, all three participating trusts approved the guidelines for use.

All midwives involved in the birth centre project were asked to read and familiarise themselves with the guidelines, a full copy of which is available in their office. Those relating to emergency procedures are also displayed on the office wall. It is likely that these will be used infrequently so it was reasoned that open display would assist midwives in being prepared to manage complications.

Guidelines brought in from Leicester Royal Infirmary also needed to be tested in their new environment. As the movement towards national guidelines gathers momentum (Baker and Fraser 1995, DOH 1997, West and Newton 1997), which seems a logical progression from a national maternity record, it was of particular interest to discern how these would be incorporated into practice in the birth centre. As local midwives had not been involved in writing them there was some curiosity surrounding perceived ownership by the users. These guidelines were quickly accepted with some minor adjustments suggesting that participation in design is not prerequisite to ownership. It appeared that when midwives were consulted about adopting these guidelines and involved in customising them for local use, they consequently 'owned' them.

Practice in an isolated setting necessitated midwives learning new skills and refreshing old ones. Midwives undertook self-analysis to identify their educational needs, and these were then addressed in a number of ways. When appropriate, updating in the consultant unit was arranged. Specialist practitioners and medical staff contributed to programmes of clinical learning, for example resuscitation, intravenous cannulation and perineal repair. Modules appropriate to identified needs of midwives were accessed through the local university, for example examination of the newborn. An interface between supervisors and providers of education is quintessential in commissioning education to meet local needs.

Experience to date in the centre is that very few women choose to give birth on a bed: the majority opt for use of water or vertical birth positions. About half elect to have a physiological third stage. Accommodation of such requests provided a challenge for midwives and gave rise to further learning needs. Midwives themselves took the initiative in filling gaps in competency by identifying and capitalising on peer expertise through workshops organised amongst themselves, thus cascading learning. It was not uncommon to find notices in the office from midwives with a particular proficiency offering support to colleagues. It quickly became evident that everyone had something to offer.

The environment is one of continuous learning and seeking to ensure the highest standards of care of mothers and babies through evidence-based decision making. Guidelines were tested in practice and care reviewed in group reflection. A midwife compared the process of development, implementation and testing of guidelines to a 'living curriculum' in education and coined the phrase, 'living guidelines' (Walker 1997, personal correspondence).

Shared learning

There is no structured programme of parenthood education. Instead, informal weekly meetings take place in the centre, attended by expectant parents and those who have given birth. Group discussions facilitated by midwives take the form of client led education. At these meetings women discuss their experiences and aspirations with carers, thus their views are taken into account. This avoids imposing routines which may lead to depersonalised care. Those who have yet to give birth identify which topics they would like covered in more depth. Midwives, students and midwifery assistants then work together to host workshops which are eagerly attended by families. Examples of topics covered are breastfeeding, alternative birthing positions and waterbirth. Postnatal women volunteer to contribute by sharing their experiences with other women, midwives, students and assistants. Women and carers learn with and from each other.

Testing boundaries of expertise

Midwives from all three trusts attend meetings held each week in the birth centre. These meetings take the form of guided reflection facilitated by a supervisor of midwives. Initially they provided a forum to test whether guidelines translated into practice. In group work it is important that each member be allowed the opportunity to contribute, to avoid polarisation through a majority view (Abraham and Shanley, 1992). It was important to agree ground rules from the outset, that anything discussed would remain confidential to the group, that the contribution of each member would be respected and valued. The aim was to arouse curiosity and encourage open debate related to care, inspiring midwives to think critically and increase personal effectiveness. As the number of deliveries was relatively small in the first few months there was opportunity to discuss each one in the context of the guidelines, thus testing whether or not they met the needs of women and professionals.

At first, some midwives tended to continue with practices rooted in hospital consultant unit experience with which they felt comfortable but which did not necessarily reflect the philosophy of the birth centre. Following discussion of one birth it was encouraging when a midwife commented, 'I didn't know that before, I think I would manage the situation differently next time'. It can be argued that the midwife develops an awareness of evidence-based practice and different options available; this empowers her in decision making to the benefit of women and their families. As the group dynamics developed, leadership was transferred to the midwives themselves, sometimes requiring a trigger from a supervisor to achieve the desired objectives.

Group reflection now focuses on issues arising from practice. These sessions provide an opportunity for midwives to debrief and learn together as the story of a birth unfolds. Midwives take turns in presenting scenarios, it may be a birth that has gone particularly well or one where complications have arisen. Peer review of record keeping is undertaken when critical analysis of the event takes place. Questions asked are: What happened here? What can be learned to repeat this success? Were there any avoidable factors and if so, what can be learned? Midwives discuss issues using the supervisor as a sounding board. They discuss the theory which informs their practice and how their practice may inform theory. They decide what needs to change in their practice to produce the most positive outcomes for families in their care. A thinking environment is promoted.

It took time for midwives to become confident in group reflection, to accept critical enquiry as non-judgmental and to trust each other in terms of confidentiality and support:

> It would be unrealistic to say that nobody's feelings are ever hurt because sometimes this causes inevitable pain. We all care deeply that what we do is right, so realising there could be a better way causes us discomfort... these are growing pains and far preferable to the anaesthetised routine that has always been good enough.
> (Midwife)

Once trust was established midwives valued reflective sessions:

> We discuss aspects of our practice knowing that we can in confidence expect unbiased and professional replies... we constantly reflect and review our practice, the guidelines and the best possible care that could have been given... this I feel is an invaluable part of the role of the birth centre as it is hopefully a forerunner of how midwifery will be practised in years to come.
> (Midwife)

The issue that most commonly emerges, in both positive and negative terms, is communication. The fifth CESDI report (DoH 1998) cited communication failures, which included poor record keeping, as factors leading to poor outcomes. The importance of effective communication, particularly when care is likely to be shared between different trusts and professionals, cannot be overemphasised.

Interpersonal relationships

Midwives from the three participating trusts accompany women from their case-load and provide care for them in the birth centre in a similar way to that in which a DOMINO scheme works. The core team midwives also have a case-load derived from women who either live out of the area or do not have a community midwife attached to their doctor's practice. A second midwife for birth, to support the core team midwife, is provided from a linked community team employed by the host trust.

In emergency situations, the consultant unit can literally be a lifeline and it is essential to preserve good working relationships. Usually the support from the receiving professionals is superb and greatly appreciated by women and midwives. The dynamics of interpersonal relationships are complicated; occasionally tensions arise and at these times it appears that midwives are not always good at caring for each other. Group reflection suggests that reasons are probably many and varied. In attempts to unravel such situations, it appears that a lack of understanding of the cultural norm established in each environment is a factor. When women undergo transfer to a consultant unit in labour they are always accompanied by their midwife who will often stay and continue as carer. In acute emergencies care is taken over by the hospital-based midwife. Relinquishing control whilst remaining an advocate for the woman has sometimes been difficult for midwives and appears to have given rise to feelings of conflict in one hospital. Hunt and Symonds (1995) suggested that considerable emotional strength was required to be an advocate for the woman when midwives recognised the potential of power and control in practice. They called this the 'agony of advocacy'. Again, communication frequently emerges as an issue in terms of what is communicated and how. Individual teams appear to achieve cohesiveness but the concept of all being part of a larger team is sometimes lacking.

These feelings need to be resolved by midwives themselves and as they become accustomed to moving between workplaces a better understanding may develop. Meetings between professional groups contribute to cognisance of the aims of personnel in managing complications particularly at a time when, however well prepared for such an event, there may be an inevitable element of disappointment for a woman as birth has not progressed as planned. Continuous effort using communication as a vehicle is ubiquitous to interprofessional working and as staff come and go, the work of all supervisors is ongoing in this area.

The centre benefits from having a named consultant obstetrician from each trust, two named general practitioners and a senior registrar in public health who act as communication links and advisers. There is an open line of communication: midwives have direct access to consultant obstetricians and paediatricians to make referrals if there is concern about the condition of mothers or babies. Except in an acute emergency, the midwife writes a letter of referral to the consultant who in turn reports the findings, management and outcome to the midwife. General practitioners are kept informed as midwives forward copies of all letters sent and received. In this way midwives are acknowledged as equal partners in care.

Credibility and 'clout'

Stapleton, Duerden and Kirkham (1998), in their research into supervision and midwifery practice, found that midwives wanted supervisors to have 'clout' within organisations. The initial named supervisor for the centre, although an experienced manager, did not have a managerial role within the organisation, neither does the current named supervisor, who is a member of the core team. In the non-hierarchical structure of the birth centre, clout within the context of managerial authority does not appear to be an issue; otherwise their expectations of their supervisor are broadly the same as reported in the above research. Midwives expect their supervisor to demonstrate leadership skills. They expect her to be knowledgeable, to acknowledge their expertise and autonomy in practice, to recognise their anxieties, to know when to act and when not to act, to communicate with appropriate people and to be assertive in negotiation. They expect advocacy on their behalf and the supervisor to be credible in the eyes of the world outside, thus credibility is 'clout'. One midwife summed up the role of the supervisor as follows:

Here the supervisor becomes a bridge… for knowledge between professionals, of communication between the birth centre and the consultant units, a bridge providing support on one's own journey through the profession. She is a source of advice and adds perspective to discussions about guidelines and helps pick a route of best practice through those situations which do not fit easily into customary practice. Although the unit has a named supervisor on whom we can all rely it also benefits from the added perspective of supervisors from the three participating consultant units who also have enthusiasm for the birth centre. (Midwife)

The role of the supervisor as a facilitator of reflection on practice and the introduction of evidence-based guidelines is acknowledged as essential in enabling midwives as confident practitioners:

The dynamic of the process is in its inclusion of the reflective discussion based in actual clinical experience, this a fundamental contribution to making the guidelines relevant to day to day practice. It also helps us as midwives to constantly reconsider our approach and management of care… It is critical that supervisors of midwives maintain a supportive profile throughout this process. We have to be 'liberated' from guidelines that dictate and restrain practice as opposed to supporting and liberating confidence in practice. (Midwife)

Midwives say they feel well supported by supervision and although they cite positive experiences of supervision in the past, they think it is even better in the birth centre. Trying to discern why this might be they concluded that whilst the nature of supervision is largely invisible, the supervisor in the workplace is visible and that gives reassurance should it be necessary to seek guidance. This would appear to have positive ramifications for a proportion of supervisors appointed from those who have a clinical role.

The value of supervision was acknowledged by the health authority when they allocated funding for the initial named supervisor to continue to provide supervisory support to the centre for a defined period of time. This was specifically to act as preceptor to a newly appointed supervisor and to continue to facilitate group reflection on practice. Such action enhances the credibility of the role.

Empowerment

Empowerment is about helping midwives to achieve their full potential; it is about expanding knowledge to give midwives confidence in their decision making. It is not something to be conferred on another, it must be released by individuals through their own self-esteem, competence and autonomy (Osterman and Kottkamp, 1993). Furneaux (1995) cites continuing education which stimulates 'critical enquiry' from the learner as pivotal to empowerment. Learning in the workplace is a cornerstone of education and a culture to which organisations should aspire (ENB 1994).

Parallels can be drawn between the empowerment of midwives and women. Confident midwives who extend the boundaries of their knowledge and practice assist women in making informed decisions about their care. The self-esteem of women is raised and they develop confidence in the ability of their own bodies and feel in control of childbirth.

Midwives had often acquired values arising from a model of managed childbirth where the professional was in control. By challenging traditions in practice through critical enquiry, they emerged as competent practitioners with confidence in physiology using guidelines underpinned by research in making evidence-based decisions. Self-development is high on the agenda and practice changes to enhance quality and meet the needs of women. A culture of lifelong learning is promoted.

> ... *women are at the centre of their care, their informed choices are paramount... we often suggest different ways we would handle situations should they recur... practising for twenty years is nothing to be proud of if it's the same year twenty times.* (Midwife)

The independent evaluation will analyse the impact of care in the birth centre on women. Results of the study cannot be foretold; however, in unsolicited comments, women report very positive experiences. They talk of being allowed to labour at their own pace, not to a clock. They speak of having confidence in the ability of their own bodies and being in control. This theme was picked up by a midwifery assistant:

> ... *women are always given an informed choice and everything is discussed. Many of them don't feel the need to make a birth plan as they are so confident that they will be given choices and make their own choices and have control of their birth... it is wonderful*

that I can see women deliver in a way that was denied to me and that every day I can finally witness changing childbirth. (Midwifery assistant)

Kirkham (1996b) wrote about the parallel processes described by Eckstein and Wallenstein (1958) applied to midwifery, that as supervisors treat midwives so midwives will treat clients. Warwick (1996) echoed this, stating that to empower women, midwives must first themselves be empowered. Experience in the birth centre has suggested that once the parallel process is initiated it becomes cyclical in nature. In the model of supervision employed, the midwife is empowered, in turn, the woman is empowered, positive feedback from women and families empowers the midwife, endorsement of the approach to practice empowers the supervisor. As long as the cycle of empowerment remains unbroken, it is self-perpetuating.

References

Abraham, C., Shanley, E. (1992). *Social Psychology for Nurses*. London: Edward Arnold.

Baker, R., Fraser, R. (1995). 'Development of review criteria: linking guidelines and assessment of quality'. *British Medical Journal* Vol. 311, pp. 370-373.

Baird, A.G., Jewell, D., Walker J.J. (1996) 'Management of labour in an isolated rural maternity hospital'. *British Medical Journal* Vol. 312, pp. 223-226.

Campbell, R., Macfarlane, A. (1994). *Where to be born? The debate and the evidence*. Oxford: National Epidemiology Unit.

Chamberlain, G., Wraight, A., Crowley, P. (eds.) (1997). *Home Births – The report of the 1994 Confidential Enquiry by the National Birthday Trust Fund*. Parthenon Publishing.

Department of Health (1992). Health Committee Second Report Session 1991-92 Maternity Services. London: HMSO.

Department of Health (1993). *Changing Childbirth*. London: HMSO.

Department of Health (1996). *Report on Confidential Enquiries into Maternal Deaths in the United Kingdom* 1991-1993. London: HMSO.

Department of Health (1997a). *The new NHS: Modern, dependable*. Government White Paper. London: HMSO.

Department of Health (1997b). (CESDI) *Confidential Enquiry into Stillbirths and Deaths in Infancy* 4th Annual Report. Maternal and Child Health Consortium. London: HMSO.

Department of Health (1998). (CESDI) *Confidential Enquiry into Stillbirths and Deaths in Infancy* 5th Annual Report. Maternal and Child Health Consortium. London: HMSO.

Dimond, B., Walters, D. (1997) *Legal Aspects of Midwifery Workbook*. Hale: Books for Midwives Press.

Dineen, M. (1997). 'Clinical risk management and midwives'. *Modern Midwife* Vol. 7, No. 11, pp. 9-13.

Eckstein, R., Wallenstein, R. (1958). *The Teaching and Learning of Psychotherapy*. New York: Basic Books.

ENB (1994). *Creating Lifelong Learners*. London: ENB.

ENB (1996). *Supervision of Midwives. The English National Board's Advice and Guidance to Local Supervising Authorities and Supervisors of Midwives*. London: ENB.

ENB (1997). *Preparation of Supervisors of Midwives. Supporting Good Midwifery Practice and Professional Development.* Module 3. London: ENB.

Flint, C. (1997). 'Midwives Will Carry the Can'. *Midwives* Vol. 110, No. 1311, p. 96.

Furneaux, N. (1995). *Achieving Professional Empowerment Through Education in Choice for the Midwife.* London: ENB.

Garcia, J., Garforth, S. (1991). 'Midwifery policies and policy-making'. In: Robinson (ed.) *Midwives, Research and Childbirth.* London: Chapman and Hall.

General Medical Services Committee (1996). *General Practitioners and Intrapartum Care: Interim Guidance.* London: BMA.

Grimshaw, J., Russell, I. (1993). 'Achieving health gain through clinical guidelines. 1: Developing scientifically valid guidelines'. *Quality in Health Care* Vol. 2, pp. 243-248.

Grimshaw, J., Eccles, M., Russell, I. (1995). 'Developing clinically valid practice guidelines'. *Journal of Evaluation in Clinical Practice* Vol. 1, No. l, pp. 37-48.

Humphris, D., Littlejohns, P. (1996). 'Implementing clinical guidelines: preparation and opportunism'. *Journal of Clinical Effectiveness* Vol. 1, No. 1, pp. 5-6.

Hundley, V.A., Cruckshank, F.M., Lang, G.D., Glazener, C.M.A., Milne, J.M., Turner, M., Blyth D., Mollison, J., Donaldson, C. (1994). 'Midwife managed delivery unit: a randomised controlled comparison with consultant led care'. *BMJ.* Vol. 309, pp. 1400-4.

Hunt, S., Symonds, A. (1995). *The Social Meaning of Midwifery.* London: Macmillan.

Hurwitz, B. (1995). 'Clinical guidelines and the law: advice, guidance or regulation?' *Journal of Evaluation in Clinical Practice* Vol. 1, No. 1, pp. 49-60.

Kirkham, M. (1996a). 'Professionalisation Past and Present: With Women or With the Powers That Be?' In: Kroll (ed.) *Midwifery Care for the Future.* London: Bailliere Tindall.

Kirkham, M. (1996b). *Supervision of Midwives.* Hale: Books for Midwives Press.

Leicester Royal Infirmary NHS Trust (1997). Evidence-Based Guidelines: Intrapartum Midwife-Led Care for Midwives.

Lewis, P., Dodd, P. (1997). 'Shoulder dystocia – drill or drama?' *Modern Midwife* Vol. 7, No. 11, pp. 30-32.

Manero, E. (1997). New Midwifery Unit in North London. *Changing Childbirth* Update No. 9.

Newdick, C. (1996). 'The status of guidelines'. *Health Care Risk Report* Vol. 2, No. 10, pp. 14-15.

Osterman, K., Kottkamp, R. (1993). 'Reflective Practice for Educators'. California Corwin Press Inc. In Furneaux, N. (1995). *Achieving Professional Empowerment Through Education in Choice for the Midwife.* London: ENB.

Price, A., Price, B. (1997). 'Making midwifery decisions'. *Modern Midwife* Vol. 7, No. 10, pp. 15-19.

Shennan, C. (1996). 'Midwives perceptions of the role of the supervisor of midwives'. In: Kirkham (ed.) *Supervision of Midwives.* Hale: Books for Midwives Press.

Stapleton, H., Duerden, J., Kirkham, M. (1998). *Evaluation of the Impact of the Supervision of Midwives on Professional Practice and the Quality of Midwifery Care.* London: ENB.

Tichy, N., Ulrich, D. (1984). 'The Leadership Challenge – A Call for the Transformational Leader'. *Sloan Management Review,* Fall 1984, pp. 59-68.

UKCC (1993). *Midwives Rules.* London: UKCC.

UKCC (1994). *The Midwife's Code of Practice.* London: UKCC.

Walker, J. (1998) 'The Edgware Birth Centre'. *MIDIRS Midwifery Digest,* Vol. 8, No. 3, pp. 376-379.

Warwick, C. (1996). 'Supervision and Practice Change at King's'. In: Kirkham M (ed.) *Supervision of Midwives.* Hale: Books for Midwives.

West, E., Newton, J. (1997). 'Clinical guidelines – An ambitious national strategy'. Editorial. *BMJ,* Vol. 315, p. 324.

Frances Derbyshire

Clinical Supervision within Midwifery

CHANGES IN PRACTICE

The neonatal unit in Exeter has 22 cots, ten of which are designated for intensive/high dependency care. The unit is staffed by a mixture of registered nurses, children's nurses, midwives and nursery nurses. Each member of the team plays a vital role in the team membership whose ultimate aim is to provide quality care for the babies it cares for and their parents. It is my belief that quality care is the fundamental right of all newborns and can be achieved only if staff are happy, motivated, knowledgeable and energized. Staff need a place where they feel able to discuss and challenge practice and be challenged. Clinical supervision holds the key.

In the document *A Vision for the Future* (DoH 1993), Yvonne Moores, Chief Nursing Officer, recommended that clinical supervision should be explored. It became target 10 of the 12 targets contained within the document for nursing, midwifery and health visiting developments.

The concept of clinical supervision is to help individuals, teams and groups to reflect on their professional activity and, by doing so, to enhance professional development, safe practice and the delivery of quality care.

Clinical supervision was introduced into the Exeter neonatal unit in January 1995 and has proved to be a valuable opportunity for staff to explore professional issues. All staff have access to clinical supervision irrespective of grade, qualification, experience or background. Clinical supervision has become firmly embodied in the culture of the unit. It is seen as useful and educative and not as a control mechanism. The term 'supervision' has connotations of control and discipline which has not always been helpful when trying to establish the purpose of supervision.

The Exeter journey to clinical supervision

Following the publication of *A Vision for the Future* the concept of clinical supervision was introduced into the Exeter neonatal unit (Derbyshire, 1997). Practising midwives had experienced 'supervision' for some time; however, it appeared to occur on an ad hoc basis for those midwives working solely in the neonatal unit. Supervisors were allocated, but access was not always easy to achieve. Practice issues, at times, appeared difficult to address within midwifery supervision as the midwifery supervisor was ill-equipped to deal with neonatal intensive care practice issues. Whilst it was crucial that practising midwives within the neonatal unit had access to midwifery supervision in line with their statutory requirement, it was clear that clinical supervision would better suit their needs within the confines of neonatology.

The implementation of clinical supervision within the unit was undertaken slowly and methodically. Information was made available for all staff in the form of articles, books and other literature. I met with every member of the team to discuss the aims of clinical supervision and gave each member of staff an information sheet. This process ensured that every member of the team was equally informed. Supervisors were identified, the prerequisites being knowledge and experience within the field of neonatology. All possessed ENB 405 and 997/998 certificates and were competent, highly skilled neonatal nurses. All had some management experience and were enthusiastic, motivated individuals, keen to develop practice and quality care. These identified supervisors were exposed to a training programme exploring group dynamics, giving and receiving feedback, listening skills, establishing contracts and safe boundaries and, most importantly, reflective practice.

Once training of supervisors had been completed, staff were asked to sign up to supervision groups. Seven groups were established. Staff had freedom of choice regarding which group to join; the only constraint was that no group should have more than eight members.

I should take time here to explain why we decided on group supervision. Clinical supervision usually takes place in a one-to-one setting or in a small group. Both have advantages and disadvantages. One-to-one supervision has the advantage of being personal highly confidential and very specific to the individual. However, it is extremely costly in terms of the amount of time required to ensure every member of staff has sufficient and regular supervision time. Group supervision is very cost-effective by comparison and has the advantage that discussions about clinical practice can be richer and more stimulating when shared among a small group of like-minded people. Group supervision allows for the exploration of issues, problem solving, recognition of others' knowledge and skills and shared learning. Provided that the groups set up contracts around confidentiality then there is no reason why very personal issues cannot be addressed within the group. On occasions it may be necessary for an individual to seek out the group supervisor for a one-to-one supervision session and this must be accommodated. However, in my experience this is rare; group supervision appears to work extremely well.

These groups have been meeting on a regular basis since June 1995. All groups decide themselves on their venue, length and frequency of meetings. Outcomes have been audited and there have been many changes in practice as a result. The groups enable staff to reflect on their professional activity and structures within their working environment. Problems in the work area are addressed and solutions found. Thinking and learning processes have been enhanced. Formal records are not kept; however, each member of the clinical supervision group is expected to undertake personal reflection and maintain a reflective journal.

Quality care/effective clinical supervision

At the beginning of this chapter I stated that it is my belief that quality care is the fundamental right of every newborn (and its parents) cared for in the neonatal unit, and that clinical supervision is the key to the success. Recent government white papers, *The New NHS: Modern, Dependable* (DoH, 1997) and *A First Class Service: Quality in the New NHS* (1998), have emphasized the need to improve the quality of care for patients. A major feature of the recent much discussed introduction of clinical governance is to guarantee quality to users of the NHS. Clinical governance is about ensuring that practice is based on scientific evidence. Until recently this has not been a feature of nursing care. The new drive to promote effective health care interventions based on evidence is an exciting one and the only sure way of delivering quality care. Evidence-based practice ensures health care professionals are confident that their interventions are informed by current and appropriate knowledge. Evidence-based practice occurs through the integration of clinical expertise with the best available external evidence from systematic research (Sackett et al, 1994).

Quality in patient care is not achieved by decree, nor by striving to reach standards set by others. Rather, it is achieved by the endless pursuit, by each individual practitioner, of greater understanding and better practice. Clinical supervision is central to this. In the Exeter neonatal unit we are fortunate to have had the vision to develop the unit to meet our needs. We have acknowledged the need for evidence-based practice and our nursing establishment now reflects our vision by supporting a research nurse post whose remit is to ensure that protocols and guidelines are evidence-based and to encourage supervision groups in their search for evidence. We also support a nurse educator post within the unit whose remit is to further develop knowledge. Gaps in knowledge are identified in supervision groups and in-service education is then addressed to ensure all unit staff have access to information. These two relatively new posts facilitate and support the health care team in gaining the necessary knowledge and skills to deliver evidence-based practice.

It would seem a nonsense to set up clinical supervision within a neonatal unit and then prevent midwives from accessing the groups simply because they already have supervision as a statutory requirement with a midwifery supervisor. They are part of the multidisciplinary team of neonatal staff and the richness of the groups is enhanced by the various experiences, knowledge and skills of the group members. Audit has proved that midwives working in the Exeter neonatal unit find participation in group clinical supervision extremely beneficial to their practice, allowing them to reflect and debate practice issues with other neonatal practitioners.

Practice and professional development

Exeter positively and actively encourages practice and professional development, ensuring that all individual health care workers in the neonatal unit have the correct knowledge, skills and competencies required for their particular field of work and contribution to the whole.

Through the research nurse post there is immediate access to information to ensure the best use of recent scientific evidence. The unit also has an excellent library and has recently obtained its own Internet link.

Supervisors of the clinical supervision groups meet regularly with myself for supervision and reflection on specific issues. This ensures that standards of care are compared to local and national standards. Areas of poor practice and potential risk are highlighted and thus standards are constantly monitored, policies and protocols written and outcomes of care audited.

Health care staff are our most valuable resource. They have the right to be valued and respected as individuals. They have the right to work in safe environments. They have the right to participate in decision making. They have the right to question procedures and practices. They have the right to appropriate education and training. In short, they have the right to clinical supervision, which will offer recognisable support and ensure the rights of individuals are met.

Clinical supervision can lead to improved staff performance and reduced rates of sickness (Kohner, 1994). Fowler (1996) states that there is no single model of supervision that can be applied uniformly across all care settings. This allows creativity amongst individuals and creativity is vital. Staff who are anxious, fearful and apathetic are not creative. We need to express creativity in our work. It is important that clinical supervision is not viewed as an imposition by the hierarchy and it is therefore important that practitioners are able to choose their own clinical supervisor and supervision group.

I am unaware of available guidelines as to how much time practitioners require for clinical supervision and therefore, when setting up clinical supervision groups, there must be a guide of what amount of time is feasible. It should be possible for any area to define what would be a reasonable maximum/minimum time requirement. This needs to be explicit in order to justify and maximise limited resources. Supervision should not encroach on personal time but should be valued as a work activity and given its place within the working rota.

All supervisors and supervisees require preparation at the outset and continued support. It is essential that some form of audit takes place but this must not be intrusive. The content of clinical supervision should remain confidential to the group. Audit should be concerned with outcomes and with detailed benefits to patient care.

Summary

Concept

Supervision helps individuals, teams and groups to reflect on their professional actions and the structures in their working environment.

Supervision helps identify solutions to problems identified in the workplace.

Supervision enhances organised thinking and learning processes.

Supervision promotes professional development, safe practice and quality care.

The guiding principle of supervision is the improvement of professional competence by a process of reflection.

The importance of implementing clinical supervision

Clinical supervision can help sustain and develop practice. It is fundamental to safeguarding standards, the development of professional expertise and the delivery of care.

The process

Every clinical practitioner should have access to clinical supervision and the process of clinical supervision should be determined by the practitioners.

There are four components to be addressed in clinical supervision:

- educative – personal development
- formative – development of skills, knowledge and advancement of safe practice
- normative – managerial component, setting standards and safe boundaries
- restorative – support, restoring health and well-being.

Contract

Clinical supervision contracts must be clear and involve:

- expectations
- goals and evaluation
- boundaries, rights and responsibilities
- methods of recording
- identifying unsafe practice and identifying appropriate action.

Rights and responsibilities

Supervisors

- establish a safe environment
- explore and clarify thinking
- give clear feedback
- share information, experiences and skills
- are aware of organisational contracts

Supervisees

- identify practice issues that need exploration or clarification
- explore interventions
- be open to feedback
- are responsible for personal development.

Conclusion

The demands that clinical supervision makes on the practice setting are considerable. Clinical supervision is particularly time-consuming if it is carried out properly. However, I believe that the Exeter neonatal experience has shown that such difficulties are far outweighed by the extensive benefits gained. The activity of clinical supervision is a major staff development activity. It enhances patient care, promotes competent, reflective practitioners and reduces stress, staff sickness and litigation. Clinical supervision should be available to all health care workers and there is no reason why midwives should be excluded.

I wish all embarking on supervision, in whatever form, enjoyment, enlightenment and fulfilment.

References

Department of Health. (1993). *A Vision for the Future. The Nursing, Midwifery and Health Visitor Contribution to Health and Health Care*. London: HMSO.

Department of Health. (1997). *The New NHS: Modern, Dependable*. London: HMSO.

Department of Health. (1998). *A First Class Service: Quality in the New NHS*. London: HMSO.

Derbyshire, F.M. (1997). '"Super-vision": Implementing Clinical Supervision in a Neonatal Unit'. *Journal of Neonatal Nursing* Vol. 3, No. 1, pp. 8-9.

Fowler, J. (1996). 'Clinical Supervision. What do you do after saying hello?' *British Journal of Nursing* Vol. 5, No. 6, pp. 382-385.

Kohner, N. (1994). *Clinical Supervision. An Executive Summary*. London: King's Fund.

Sackett, L.D., Rosenburg, W., Haynes, B.R. (1997). *Evidence-based Medicine: How to Practise and Teach EBM*. London: Churchill Livingstone.

Anonymised Case Studies
of Supervisory Practice

CASE STUDY 1

This case study is written by the midwife and supervisor concerned. The names have been changed to ensure anonymity but they wish it to be known that they are in the West Midlands. The new West Midlands LSA guidance document is attached to this case study at the request of the supervisor and LSA concerned.

THE MIDWIFE'S STORY:
My involvement with the birth of my grandchild

In January this year, my daughter Sarah gave birth to an 8lb 6oz baby boy in the birthing pool at X Hospital. It was a beautiful birth and Sarah and the baby were discharged after six hours. I cared for Sarah throughout the postnatal period and she did not see any other midwives during this time. The baby was fully breastfed.

Sarah had said from the beginning of pregnancy that she wanted me to look after her during labour. She had originally planned to have a home birth but her partner Gordon was fearful about this, believing that it would be safer for the baby to be born in hospital. I tried to reassure him by explaining what is known about the safety of home birth but towards the end of her pregnancy, Sarah's blood pressure rose slightly and she was admitted to hospital overnight. This strengthened Gordon's belief that the baby should be born in hospital.

In view of this, I went to see my supervisor of midwives to ask if I would be permitted to look after her during labour. My supervisor discussed the matter with the consultant under whose care Sarah was booked and it was agreed that I could look after my daughter. The only proviso was that if labour and delivery did not proceed normally and there were any decisions to be made about management of care, I should consult with another midwife.

A friend who is a midwife at the same unit agreed to put herself on call and when the time came, she came into the unit to help us. As I have said, the baby was born under water and it was actually the other midwife who lifted him from the water and passed him to me whilst she cut his cord. Although I did examine Sarah in early labour, as labour progressed, I acted more as a doula (Walters and Kirkham, 1997) than a midwife.

I was grateful that my supervisor agreed to my involvement with Sarah's care. Several colleagues have expressed the view that with her first baby, my daughter was 'lucky' to have had such an easy labour and delivery. I am positively convinced that this was because I was able to love, cherish and look after her throughout her labour.

THE SUPERVISOR'S STORY:
Proactive midwifery supervision

Background

Mary is a recently qualified midwife who is an enthusiastic practitioner with maturity, common sense and an extraordinary empathy with pregnant women, making her an extremely effective advocate.

At the commencement of her employment we met to discuss her needs in respect of a preceptor and placement in this establishment which provided fairly traditional midwifery care.

Some months later, Mary approached me with her news that her daughter, Sarah, was pregnant and that this was to be her first grandchild. Sarah had asked that her mother be allowed to care for her, particularly during labour, and to give her all her postnatal care. Mary was very keen to gain my consent and support as her daughter was booked under the care of a hospital consultant.

Views regarding delivering close friends and family are many and varied and in fact the two managers/supervisors in this maternity unit have opposite views.

Discussion

During this time we talked about Mary's clinical skills, her ability to function in an emergency and the difficulties surrounding caring for someone with whom she is emotionally involved.

The agreement

- Mary would book annual leave to ensure that she would be available.

- A midwife supporter on labour ward would be selected by Mary who would oversee care given, help in decision making if needed and be present at the delivery as second midwife.

- I would make myself available at any time to give advice and support.

- Mary would inform me when Sarah was safely delivered.

- I would speak to Sarah's consultant regarding our arrangements.

Following our discussion I met with the consultant obstetrician and got the distinct impression that he was not happy with the plan. His view was that it was unwise to give direct care to one's close relatives. I reminded him that as a manager of the service and a supervisor of midwives, I was responsible for the provision of midwifery care and assured him that we had a strategy for ensuring safe, appropriate care for his patient. There were no further objections following this clarification.

Outcome

Sarah was safely delivered of a healthy baby, her care in labour went as planned with Mary fully supported by a senior midwife. Mary also provided all the postnatal care at home, informing the supervisor of midwives of her intention to practise in her area.

Reflection

Later that week, Mary and I held an informal debrief over the telephone and we were both pleased with the way events had progressed. I was always confident of Mary's capabilities and felt reassured by our forward planning. I felt that supervision was carried out in a supportive manner, aware of the pitfalls of being heavy handed or prescriptive.

West Midlands Local Supervising Authority Consortium

Regional guidance for supervisors of midwives when receiving requests from midwives to deliver relatives or friends

1. Introduction

1.1 Whilst it is recognised that all midwives are accountable for their practice in whatever environment they are practising (UKCC, 1998), experience has shown that midwives who care for their friends and relatives in labour (including colleagues), need to consider the potential for increased stress and emotional involvement which may hinder objective decision-making and therefore they may require additional support and guidance.

1.2 Supervisors have an important contribution to make by ensuring that midwives fully understand the implications and by ensuring that appropriate support and guidance is provided.

1.3 This guidance is not intended to limit the sphere of practice of the midwife or to be an obstacle to the midwife's ability to provide midwifery care to a relative or friend.

1.4 It is, however, important that the midwife practitioner understands and acknowledges the potential conflict and possible pressures looking after relatives or friends may engender.

2. Process

2.1 Receipt of written request as early as possible in pregnancy from the woman with supporting written statement from the midwife proposing to deliver. (This request would normally be addressed to the manager who should involve the supervisor at this point.)

2.2 The supervisor should arrange an appointment with the midwife to discuss the support and guidance required (see checklist).

2.3 The discussion should be informal with the emphasis on the role of the supervisor of midwives as supporter to the midwife. Documentation of discussion to be copied to the midwife and retained in the supervisor's file.

2.4 The supervisor may also wish to visit the woman to discuss her reasons for the request and the possible implications.

2.5 Recommendation to management to either support or not support the request, with reasons.

2.6 Request to management to enable appropriate updating and support to be provided.

2.7 Notify colleague supervisors of arrangements.

2.8 Post-delivery review session with midwife.

Checklist of principles to be considered

1 Does the midwife appear happy to care for the woman or has she been pressurised into agreeing?

2 Does the midwife recognise that the emotional involvement will increase the stress associated with the delivery? What strategies has she got in place to cope with the additional stress?

3 Is the midwife familiar with practising in the chosen environment... i.e. hospital/community, a different trust? Does she need an honorary contract?

4 Has the midwife had up to date experience of working on the delivery suite or conducting a home delivery (as appropriate)? Does she need an orientation programme? Is she eligible to practise? Has she submitted a NOITP?

5 Is the midwife fully conversant with local policies/protocols/ procedures?

6 Does the midwife require any updating to enable her to practise competently, e.g. normal labour, water birth, home birth, abnormal labour, interpretation of CTGs etc.?

7 Are there any risk factors? Is the woman considered to be within a low or high risk category?

8 Is the midwife able to allocate time for the client while continuing with her present workload? Has she discussed off-duty/leave arrangements?

9 Is the midwife happy to accept support from another experienced midwife (a "buddy") when the woman is in labour and during the delivery? This is to protect the midwife and not to undermine her professional autonomy.

10 Does the woman accept the presence of the second midwife? Does she realise that the midwife will have to hand over her care if the labour is prolonged and the midwife is in danger of becoming over-tired? Does the midwife acknowledge her own limitations?

11 Where a hospital delivery is planned, does the midwife accept that the labour suite co-ordinator will oversee the progress of the labour (as part of her role and in addition to the 'buddy' midwife)?

12 Does the midwife accept that the 'buddy' as well as the co-ordinator may challenge decisions where the midwife's objectivity or practice is in question?

13 Has the supervisor arranged to meet the midwife following the delivery in order to reflect on the experience?

CASE STUDY 2

The narrative which follows is drawn from the transcripts of an interview between a supervisor and a midwife following a critical incident whereby IM Pethidine and Syntometrine were given to a woman in established labour. The names of the midwives have been changed, as have any features which might otherwise identify individuals or the maternity unit concerned.

THE MIDWIFE'S PERSPECTIVE

The setting

Kathleen worked as a G grade integrated midwife in a large, inner city teaching hospital. She was an experienced practitioner who, when covering the labour ward, was often the most senior midwife on duty. Her career, spanning almost 20 years and interrupted only for maternity breaks, had been without serious incident or complaint. Kathleen had taken care of her own professional development for many years and was up to date with refresher requirements at the time of the incident. She had recently completed a university degree in a non-midwifery subject.

The maternity unit served a mixed ethnic and white working class population. It was a friendly and progressive unit and had made great efforts to tailor care in a way which was sensitive to the needs of all service users. The midwives were 'doggedly' enthusiastic about their work and thought themselves fortunate to be employed by a trust which was working towards recognising the needs of employees and supporting a no-blame culture. Midwifery supervision in the unit was perceived by some midwives as a helpful and supportive mechanism. Cross-supervision (i.e. separation of the managerial and supervisory roles) had been in place for some time.

The prelude

It was late in the afternoon of a cold, wet January day. K was on call and had just returned home after finishing her busy antenatal clinic. She was looking forward to a cup of tea and a cigarette. The clinic had run late because one of her clients had needed referral for an obstetric consultation and another had needed consoling because her teenage daughter had just been suspended from school. Just as K was shedding her coat and kicking off her shoes, the phone rang. A colleague on another team asked her to go to the labour ward to take over the care of a woman in established labour. The midwife on call for this team already had two clients in labour and the second on call had just phoned in with a migraine. K sighed, pulled her coat back on, looked longingly at the teapot, grabbed a couple of apples and locked the door of her flat behind her.

Rush hour traffic more than doubled the journey time to the unit but it also allowed K a little breathing space in which to leave the worries of the day behind and to prepare herself for a busy night ahead. She arrived on the labour ward shortly after 1800hrs. The labour ward was humming with activity. It had been an exceptionally busy day and an emergency section was under way. Two women were awaiting epidurals. A midwifery colleague greeted K and briefly introduced her to the client (M).

The incident

K had not previously met M or her partner. She described them as ' non-English and non-white'. Both sets of parents had immigrated from Africa and although both M and her partner had been born and educated in England, K sensed 'there would be many cultural differences'. She was on her guard, forming a hunch that, although nothing had been said, M's partner 'was on the lookout for trouble… that he'd obviously been the victim of much… that he was on the lookout for racism and problems'.

This was M's first baby. Her pregnancy had followed a normal pattern and she had started labour spontaneously and at term. She had started contracting at 0600hrs that morning. The presentation of the baby was cephalic, the lie longitudinal with the vertex deeply engaged. The previous vaginal examination had revealed that M's cervix was 5cm dilated with intact membranes. A CTG was in progress; M was contracting well and the foetal heart was reactive.

M was distressed with the contractions but in between them 'she was absolutely fine… she was wanting to eat crisps and things… I felt she could be easily calmed and helped through them but the partner was panicking… he was much more distressed by her pain than she was. He was insisting that she should have an epidural'. K tried to show M how to use the entonox 'but it was a bit too late… it should have been done earlier but nobody had had the time. She couldn't relax… she was still panicking at the beginning of every contraction and her partner was getting quite aggressive and kept insisting that an epidural was what she needed'. K could not find a birthplan in M's notes and M could not recall having made one. Following a brief, but futile, attempt to elicit her preferences for her labour and birth, K gave in to the pressure and called the anaesthetist, only to find she was still in OT and two clients were already awaiting an epidural ahead of M. K suggested M try Pethidine as an interim measure. She explained that the use of Pethidine 'was something I rarely do because I don't like it but when we have somebody where relaxation is such a problem it can help. I discussed the pros and cons with both of them and I do mean discussed, because these two, her partner in particular, had obviously heard bad stories about either our particular unit or... he was on the lookout for trouble. So it was quite a lengthy discussion.'

K continued her recall of the events: 'I checked the Pethidine and an antiemetic... You know what it's like on busy units on a Sunday, we'd run out of absolutely everything. I had to search for everything, nothing was immediately available because nobody had had time to restock. There weren't any kidney dishes in the stock cupboard so I grabbed one from another room, put the Pethidine and the antiemetic into it and asked the other midwife to give me the Syntometrine from the fridge next door. I thought I'd get them all at once in case M made rapid progress and I didn't have time to come out again. Labour ward was busy so I couldn't guarantee that a second midwife would be present. I was trying to look ahead and be well prepared.'

K went on to say that even as she put the Syntometrine with the other two drugs, she was aware that this was not a good idea and resolved to separate them as soon as she returned to M's room. On the way back, K remembered that M was without an ID band so she stopped to remedy this. By the time she had finished, the second midwife who had checked the Pethidine and Syntometrine with K had been called back to her own client and there was nobody else around. K checked the ID band with M and her partner and proceeded to give M what she thought was the Pethidine, together with the antiemetic. K then put the empty phials, needle and syringes into the sharps bin. At this point K realised, to her horror, that the unopened phial in the kidney dish was not syntometrine but the antiemetic. She had given M Syntometrine and Pethidine. K's immediate response was to ring the emergency bell and 'unbelievingly to give the antiemetic as well thinking, oh my god, if she's not sick now she's going to be in a minute…'. In the few minutes before help arrived, K tried to explain what had happened to M and her partner.

The registrar was with M within 5 minutes of the injection having been administered. M was immediately transferred to OT and an emergency LSCS performed. A midwife colleague assisted K who described herself as 'being completely numb… I was so frightened… I just thought the baby was going to die'. The baby was born in excellent condition with apgars of 7, 9 and 10.

More high dependency women than usual had been admitted to the labour ward over the previous 24 hours and this had left stocks depleted and staff feeling stretched to capacity. In the circumstances, K felt it inappropriate to hand over the care of M to an unknown colleague so she stayed with M and her partner throughout the night. She also decided to wait and see her supervisor (L) before going off duty the following morning. K was appalled by what had happened and 'although I appreciated it was very serious, it was also a complete mistake. It was an unforgivable human error but it was a human error. I knew I could be sacked for this; I could lose my job and be struck off. But I wasn't panicking about that because it didn't really sink in… I was actually quite calm. You know that calm that's not really calm, there's a volcano underneath but you turn it off until later.'

Colleagues' responses to the incident

K described her supervisor as being '… exemplary really, in terms of what you would expect from a supervisor under the circumstances. I felt totally supported. By that I mean she let me talk through it even though by this time I'd been up a long time and really needed to go home. I was just gabbling. I wasn't making much sense but she let me do that and it calmed me down. She picked up the salient points of what had happened and told me that, from what she'd heard, it sounded like I had made a serious mistake. That it was a very serious incident and that it would be investigated but that it seemed like a genuine human error which I had realised quickly and done all the right things afterwards. She told me I should go home and try not to panic. She asked me if I needed anybody with me and said that she'd see me the first thing next morning and we'd go through it again together and write it all down. She made me feel that she was concerned about me. She was concerned that I went home and got a rest before I started to write a report. She was very, very good at her job. I know I was very lucky to have her as my supervisor.' K confided that, apart from an annual supervisory review, she had never 'had dealings with supervisors before... not since the old days when the supervisor was just the enemy and that was that'.

K volunteered that the support she received from her midwife colleagues immediately after the incident was 'completely wonderful... they backed me up and helped me out. They were all very calm. Thinking back, it was what I would have expected and what I would have given to them in return. But I was still very grateful for the midwives who were around that evening. It could have been different if other midwives had been on.'

The following day, K discussed her supervisor's response with a close midwifery colleague who warned her against 'being so relaxed about it... she told me I should stay on my guard... that dreadful things can still happen to you even though you're being reassured... that I shouldn't automatically trust the supervisor just because she listened to me and sympathised with me. She was warning me about being too confident in L... that someone could pull the rug if I was too laid back about it all.'

In mitigation

By way of mitigating circumstances, K explained that she had been 'having terrible financial problems at the time and over this period they all came to a head. For one reason or another I was off sick. Thinking back though, I don't think I would have done it any differently if I had been L except that I think I'd have left the midwife more time to write the essay so that it didn't seem like a punitive thing. It took me a surprisingly long time to recover from the shock. I know that she didn't mean the essay as a punishment, but that's how it felt. But I have to say that I think the supervision in this instance, in my case, was as good as it gets in my experience of midwifery.'

ACTION TAKEN

Managerial

An internal investigation was carried out immediately by the hospital trust management. This was usual practice for any serious incident, regardless of whether the incident was a 'near miss' or, as with this case, had actually happened. L, who had been a midwifery manager for three years, was asked to take the role of investigating officer. As a result of the investigation, the drug administration procedure was reviewed and the attention of all labour ward staff was drawn to the correct procedure. The keys to the theatre lifts were made more accessible and all labour ward staff were made aware of the security code for the operating theatre suite.

Supervisory

As stated, the only investigation into this incident was instigated by the hospital trust management. The investigating officer (L) was a midwifery supervisor whose authority and leadership within the unit commanded widespread respect. At the time of the incident, L had been K's named supervisor but as soon as she was asked to undertake the investigation, L made provision for a supervisor colleague whom K knew and trusted, to provide supervisory support. The supervisory action included a request that K attend a risk management study day of her choice and write a 5,000 word essay on an associated topic.

K's response to the verdict 'was a huge relief... I thought I'd be suspended. I just thought that's what happens in these cases... I felt that that judgement was very fair. I had made a bad mistake which shouldn't have happened and I needed to look at the way it had happened to make sure it didn't happen again. So it was fair and I was quite enthusiastic about the thought of doing it but after a few days I started to feel like a naughty schoolgirl being given an essay to write... So I thought it was fair and it was appropriate but all the same, I did wonder when the flaming heck am I going to have time to do it.'

Colleagues' responses to the action taken

K was of the opinion that some of her midwifery colleagues 'thought I'd got off really lightly but others thought much the same as me; that I'd been given a hundred lines to do. But the verdict itself, we thought that was fair and reasonable and L was at pains to explain that it wasn't by way of a punishment, it was by way of getting something positive out of it. I'd been picking her brains anyway about a module I'd been doing about supervision... we'd been talking to each other about writing about supervision anyway, as part of my personal development, so I'm sure she saw it as a continuation of that. That's how I saw it too really. I knew that was how she meant it but it did still feel a bit like being given an essay to write.'

One year on

K has not yet attended the study day and nor has she written the essay. L is about to leave her present job. K stated that she has 'no intention of doing the essay... I object to the fact that she [L] will not take on that I really have learned from this experience without it [the essay]. I've got enough overtime hours already and I'm not adding to them by doing essays in my own time!'

THE SUPERVISOR'S PERSPECTIVE

The context and purpose of investigating a critical incident

L described her employing trust as promoting 'a culture of openness that's been there right from the beginning'. This contrasted with the trust for whom she had previously worked where the unwritten rule was 'never admit to being at fault'. She found this to be 'an untenable position which I think actually increased the potential for litigation'. The experience gained in her present post had convinced L of the need for all midwives to see accountability as 'something everyday and real. It's things like writing statements, challenging the medical staff when they're making decisions which are not in women's interests... things like that... They begin to see that these things are not so frightening... that committing something to paper about their practice is simply part of the process of being accountable and not about being fearful or feeling inappropriately responsible.' This philosophy of openness and accountability guided the process of fact finding and subsequent hearing for any critical incident in the trust.

L was of the opinion that critical incidents didn't 'just happen' and that only rarely could fault be attributed to 'any one person's failings on one isolated occasion'. This rationale influenced the entire investigation, including the manner in which the facts were collected and the evidence was presented. The process of fact finding needed to include 'everything possible... if you're talking about potential litigation then what you don't want is a solicitor phoning you up two or ten years down the line and asking for evidence you never thought to collect. That's why the process of investigation has to be given time... to get as many facts as possible from everyone concerned... You need that time to make it harder for people to jump to conclusions or make quick judgements... So you need to meet with people... you need to meet them with empathy and understanding because asking people to write statements about painful events is not easy... you need to find out if there were any mitigating circumstances... what the staffing levels were like, for example. Basically, you need to make your case as robust as possible so that when any decisions are made, they come from the evidence and not from someone's prejudice... You have to remember that you're not there to act as judge or jury, you're there to find and present the facts and look at these against current standards of practice and against what common sense might dictate. If you find that, despite a bad outcome, everyone involved performed well and in line with our current state of knowledge and evidence, then fine, you've got nothing else to say... but you have to remember that the parents and even other colleagues will see it differently... they'll more than likely be wanting to blame someone so you have to do all you can to help them through that tendency.'

L explained that the process of investigating a critical incident usually identified a number of features which needed to be changed in order to reduce the chances of the incident recurring and to ensure that the care being given was more effective. Values such as transparency and honesty guided the investigation process, making it unlikely that a 'cover-up' would be tolerated. L was of the opinion that 'cover-ups' did happen, especially where trust management did not respect their employees. L thought that this attitude worked against both the welfare of service users and the credibility of the organisation.

'When there's a cover-up and I really mean a cover-up, you're no longer serving or caring for those people... you're also potentially increasing their psychological morbidity because when people aren't given honest answers, then they become angry and vengeful... it causes a lot of distrust. People can smell a mile off when something isn't being said which should be being said. And what does that do for the reputation of the trust, especially if they need to use the health services again? And what message does it send from management or the corporate side to the clinicians? So the process by which we do things... like critical incident investigation is really, really important because that's one way we can bring home to everyone that changing the culture can make a difference. It's about being honest and saying that nobody can guarantee a particular outcome... It's starting with that and helping people to accept that.'

The skills required to undertake an investigation

L reminded me that she had not investigated this incident in the role of K's supervisor; that had been temporarily taken over by a colleague. The skills L cited as being important to the process of investigation were those of: 'critical reflection, absolute clarity, lateral thinking, a strong sense of fairness... being systematic and very methodical'. It required her to meet with and talk to absolutely anybody who might have been involved; a facility for minute detail such as noting what the weather was like on the day, the state of the unit equipment, sickness levels, staffing levels and expertise; perhaps even looking at other women's notes. 'And then you have to put it all in context... It's exhausting and it's pretty time-consuming... It's a really time-hungry exercise. But the consequences of getting it wrong, I couldn't live with ...'

One characteristic L felt was out of place in the supervisory relationship was that of friendship: 'When people say the supervisor needs to be your friend, I find that difficult to go along with. There are times when friendship really gets in the way of a relationship like that. You can have empathy, you can have an enabling attitude, you can look at the support system that person needs and you can develop good listening skills, but one thing it sure ain't is friendship. It's way beyond that...'

The initial fact finding exercise

L made her preliminary enquiries and concluded that this was 'a cut and dried case – it's happened. It was a serious incident but the midwife responded immediately and the appropriate action was taken. The baby was absolutely fine but the mother did have surgery and potentially unnecessary surgery as far as anyone could tell.'

The process of investigation

This unit has incorporated a process of review into the investigation proceedings as a preliminary to reaching a final verdict. All those involved in the incident will be invited to come together and review the case and the evidence. The need for confidentiality is emphasised and everyone is given a set of the casenotes. The consultant for the woman concerned usually chairs the panel. L said: 'I've come to realise that it really does matter how that meeting is chaired... it really can influence the decisions which are made so we're looking at that quite closely... But on the whole, it's been really positive and the feedback I've had from the individuals involved is that they have appreciated it... it's helped them to integrate the experience and made them feel more supported going back to the clinical environment. But we're still experimenting with it... There is a difference between meeting people on their own and meeting them in a group situation and then of course there's a difference in the multidisciplinary setting... At the beginning it was always... it was almost an unspoken rule that midwives can't judge doctors... In this case some of the doctors did feel that maybe a suspension or something else should have happened... It's taken some of them a while to appreciate that as an investigating officer you're not judging... What we're encouraging everyone to recognise is that the organisation needs to change... and what we're suggesting is that nurturing a sense of the individual being accountable and open is what it's all about... it's also about those individuals – especially midwives – not feeling inappropriately responsible...'

L volunteered that 'Some of the things which came out of that process were memos and a report to all midwives about the administration of drugs. So it didn't end up all being focused on K because some of the issues were about what I call custom and practice. For instance, the other midwife should have gone in with K and checked the administration of the Pethidine but she didn't...'

A copy of the proceedings from the review process is sent to the Chief Executive and a response is always made. L emphasised the need for feedback at every level of the organisation and maintained that this was possible. She was, however, concerned about maintaining the confidentiality of those involved because, 'When something like this happens, you've no control over the whisper factory. I'm not at liberty to share the findings of the investigation or the hearing and neither should I; there is no reason why anyone should know what happened. Of course everyone knows if someone is suspended but if they're not, then they're not going to necessarily know that a person is going through a set of learning objectives for example...'

Outcome and recommendations

As described earlier, K was given a learning contract which included attending a risk management study day and writing a 5,000 word essay on a related topic. Neither of these tasks have been achieved and L is now wondering whether the 'softly softly' approach was appropriate. L was aware at the time that 'this particular lady was in quite a stretched place in her personal life and had been for some time and she was completely aware of that herself. I have to take that into account but she's still in that place... so how long can that go on for?... It feels like unfinished business... I don't think it's appropriate that she doesn't achieve the learning objectives but I'll be moving on from this job soon and I'd like to see it completed. I know there's no point in overloading her or asking the impossible but part of me is saying, Hang on a minute, that still needs to be done. I feel that K has the capacity and I felt that she would benefit from learning about the organisational side of practice. I actually thought that the nice bit of this learning process was to go to a clinical study day and when she didn't go I was a bit pissed off about it. We both looked at what was available in the college but decided the standard wasn't... But this was state of the art stuff... it was really good stuff but she ended up not going and she didn't tell me either... I know it was part and parcel of what was happening for her at that moment but I also think it was salutary and there's a little bit of dis-ease in me about it... We all go through difficult places in our lives but if it goes on and on then it's bound to impact on your work...'

L confided that 'supervising someone through the process of a learning contract is hard work because it means pressing that person to engage at a different level and to embed the learning a bit more at a practice level. The learning process isn't just about saying, Oh dear, I really didn't mean to do it... I wanted K to understand that this incident was reflecting a particular pattern of poor practice... We needed to look at why she was cutting corners... how she came to be in a position where it was possible to mix scheduled drugs up in a kidney dish. It's about getting her to appreciate the need for a framework to protect her against the human error factor... It's all part of preventing against the sloppy practice that goes on all the time... Sometimes critical incidents bring our attention to the fact that it's the little factors that keep getting missed which finally tip the balance... But I'm as concerned about the morbidity as I am about the mortality aspect of care and that's much more pervasive and it's much harder to change because it's not usually very visible. But that's what I think we should be tackling in supervision... we need to start defining some of the issues ourselves rather than have, say, the CESDI report telling us...'

For the future

L was very excited about continuing to develop in her role as a supervisor. Her new job would mean less time in the clinical environment but she felt this would more than be compensated for by new skills she would be learning. She sees this as a new opportunity to tackle some of the issues around poor practice because, 'The same things keep coming up everywhere, whether it's from investigations like this or from CESDI... it's consistently commenting on poor practice, on bad supervision, poor communication and poor people management. I think there's something that we haven't untwigged yet and I think it's about relationships. I don't think I've got the skills to deal with the issues involved... The supervisors' course didn't really touch on that... I remember we had quite a good session on interviews and listening skills and a reasonable one on report writing but the rest of it was a bit duff really. I think it is possible to make these big changes but I don't think we have the skills yet... not in supervision anyway.'

CASE STUDY 3

Pauline had been working on night duty in a busy city hospital for 15 years. She was happy on nights, it suited her family and meant she could organise her home life with minimum disruption. She had been encouraged to rotate on to days to broaden her midwifery experience by her manager and supervisor but had resisted this strongly and, supported by her union steward, successfully.

Pauline didn't like the idea of day duty. She didn't like the day staff and felt there was an atmosphere between night and day staff. She felt more secure, and less intimidated, at night. She didn't need to get involved in 'trust politics', neither did she want to go on study days when she was content to attend a refresher course every five years. It was a bit of an upheaval leaving the family, but they coped, and it was a nice change for her.

So Pauline continued until a complaint was made about her. The couple concerned, Mr and Mrs Smith, alleged that Pauline had been unsupportive on the telephone and uncaring on admission. They said she demonstrated a lack of urgency or concern as Mrs Smith's labour had progressed. No poor practice, as such, was reported, but Pauline's attitude had allegedly marred Mrs Smith's birth experience significantly.

Pauline was devastated. There had never been any other complaints made about her and she wasn't aware that any of her colleagues felt her work was below standard. The trust set up a formal inquiry into the complaint and Pauline was encouraged to seek the support of her named supervisor of midwives, Elspeth. The delivery suite manager and supervisor of midwives conducted the inquiry and found various record keeping errors on Mrs Smith's notes with substantial gaps in care. As a result, several other sets of Pauline's notes were reviewed and found to be of poor quality. These were shared with Elspeth.

Pauline met with Elspeth and they discussed the various issues which had been highlighted by the complaint and case note review. Elspeth explained to Pauline that her role was to support Pauline, as her named supervisor, and in this role her responsibility was to the LSA and Pauline and not to the trust. The delivery suite manager was acting on behalf of the trust.

After much discussion, when Elspeth was able to highlight which aspects of the *Midwives Rules and Code of Practice* (UKCC, 1998) had been breached and which aspects of the *Guidelines for Practice* (UKCC ,1996) had not been followed, Pauline began to realise that she had begun to let her practice slide. Her original denial and anger, following this opportunity for reflection, began to wane and be replaced by a realisation that she had made mistakes and she expressed her desire to improve her practice and get 'back on track'.

Elspeth prepared a supervisory learning contract for Pauline, which involved a period of supervised practice, supported by Elspeth, which would embrace all the aspects of learning identified by the investigation. Pauline realised that she was out of touch with many midwifery developments and agreed to work on days throughout the supervisory support programme. This programme involved working for a period of time in all areas of the maternity unit and included a period on community. Record keeping workshops and ENB approved study days relating to accountability were planned.

Pauline worked with a preceptor in each new area and met with Elspeth every week to review her progress and reflect on new learning. In the first few days Pauline had been very apprehensive and some of her old defences emerged, but gradually she settled down and began to enjoy midwifery again.

Meanwhile, the trust had instigated a disciplinary hearing as a result of the complaint. Elspeth acted as Pauline's advocate, detailing the supervisory support programme and Pauline's positive response. The panel decision was to support the supervision programme and not take any disciplinary action.

Pauline grew in confidence throughout the programme and became eager to learn more. She enlisted Elspeth's support in accessing a module on the A26 diploma programme and this was willingly given as Pauline was achieving all the learning outcomes identified on her supervisory learning contract.

At the end of the supervisory support programme Elspeth was delighted to sign the learning contract indicating that all learning outcomes had been achieved.

Pauline never returned to permanent nights. She now rotates her shifts with the rest of her colleagues and was recently awarded an F grade.

References

UKCC (1996). *Guidelines for Practice*. London: UKCC.

UKCC (1998). *Midwives Rules and Code of Practice*. London: UKCC.

Walters, D. and Kirkham, M.J. (1997) 'Support and control in labour: doulas and midwives'. In: Kirkham, M.J. (ed.) Perkins, E.R. (ed.) *Reflections on Midwifery*. London: Ballière Tindall.

Glynnis Mayes

Development of the
New Open Learning Programme

EDUCATION FOR SUPERVISORS

In June 1997 the English National Board for Nursing, Midwifery and Health Visiting (ENB) launched the new open learning programme for the preparation of supervisors of midwives. The programme was developed from the previous pack published by the ENB which had undergone a major revision. Statutory supervision of midwives had been developing rapidly since the first open learning programme was introduced four years earlier, and the programme was updated in order to:

- reflect recent changes in legislation
- equip supervisors of midwives to contribute to the current health service developments
- offer insights into the potential of supervision of midwives for developing midwifery practice.

The revised and updated programme was developed to meet the needs of midwives who had been nominated for appointment as supervisors of midwives. The focus of the programme was on developing a proactive approach to supervision which supports midwives in all areas of practice as accountable practitioners and which contributes to meeting local and national objectives such as clinical audit and risk management. The open learning programme had been designed as the theoretical component for incorporation in the ENB R68 programme 'Preparation for Supervisors of Midwives', although it has been used as a valuable resource in a range of different situations.

Background

Supervision of midwives has been in existence since the Midwives Act of 1902 established the framework for the professional regulation of midwives in England and Wales. Throughout the intervening years there have been major changes in the context in which midwives have practised and the characteristics of the maternity services have undergone regular transformation, but supervision of midwives has survived. It was not until 1993 that formal preparation for the role as a qualification for appointment as a supervisor was introduced, a relatively recent development in the lifespan of supervision.

The first statutory educational requirement pertaining to supervision was the five-yearly refresher course. This was specified in the *Rules of the Central Midwives Board* (CMB) issued in 1939 for those midwives who were employed as non-medical supervisors of midwives. No preparation for the role was required and nor were the supervisors required to notify their intention to practise. This is curious in the light of the regulations issued in the Ministry of Health Circular of 1937, concerning the role and expectations of supervisors of midwives. The circular emphasises the importance of appointing supervisors who 'have adequate experience in the practice of midwifery' and who 'not only possess the necessary professional qualifications, but who also have the essential qualities of sympathy and tact' (Ministry of Health 1937, Circular 1620).

Forty years later, these regulations were superseded by a new statutory instrument which specified the qualifications of supervisors of midwives (SI no. 1580, 1977). All supervisors of midwives were required to be practising midwives and the category for medical supervisors was abolished. Supervisors were now required to attend an induction course approved by the CMB, within six months of appointment. As a result, the first induction courses for supervisors of midwives were introduced by the CMB in 1978. They consisted of two days initially, and were extended later to three days, when the responsibility for provision was transferred to the ENB in 1983. There was still no educational preparation prior to taking on the role, and newly appointed supervisors were left to seek guidance from colleagues as the need arose. There was therefore little consistency in either the perception of the role or what supervisors actually did. For the most part this consisted of the administrative tasks of processing statutory notifications, or intervening when midwives deviated from the supervisors' views of safe practice (Jenkins 1995, Kirkham 1995).

The first programmes of preparation for supervisors

By the early 1990s the ENB had developed a strategy for strengthening supervision of midwives and enhancing its effectiveness, in collaboration with the officers of the local supervising authority (LSA). Included within the strategy was the introduction of a structured educational programme as a mandatory prerequisite for the appointment as a supervisor of midwives in England. An innovative feature of the programme was the use of open learning as the vehicle for midwives to acquire the skills and knowledge essential for the role. This offered a learner centred, work based approach to meet the diverse needs and circumstances of the midwives nominated and selected to become supervisors of midwives.

The Board commissioned the production of open learning materials as the core text for the preparation of supervisors of midwives (ENB, 1992) The materials were incorporated into ENB approved programmes delivered in five centres throughout England. Essential components of the programmes included:

- completion of the open learning programme
- attendance at study days at the course centre
- mentorship from an experienced supervisor
- academic support from a midwifery tutor counsellor
- assessment at the level of diploma in higher education
- attendance at an ENB study day at the end of the programme.

The open learning programme was developed at a time when there was very little published on supervision of midwives, and there were many inconsistencies in the practice and interpretation of the role. It was necessary therefore to ensure that the ENB publication reflected not only the legislation but also sound professional input. The work was undertaken involving the midwifery officers of the ENB, members of the Midwifery Committee and expert authors, recognised for their expertise and achievements associated with supervision of midwives. The final publication was informed by the comments of the critical readers and by the experiences of midwives who worked through the draft programme in the developmental testing stage.

The aim of the open learning programme was to enable prospective supervisors of midwives to gain the understanding and the knowledge nesessary to take on the responsibilities of the role. It was produced as four separate modules in the style of open learning to address the essential components of supervision:

- The statutory basis to the role of the supervisor
- The role of the supervisors in supporting good midwifery practice
- The role and responsibility of the supervisor in dealing with alleged professional misconduct
- The supervisor's role in professional development.

For the first time, there was a substantive text available for reference by all supervisors which promoted a clear approach and set the standard for supervision throughout the country.

The open learning programme was evaluated by the Board in 1995 by exploring the experiences of the users who had worked through the pack. Data was collected by means of nominal group evaluation by 104 midwives in eight groups, and interviews with 20 participants from two course centres. All participants were very positive about the programme even though some had completed it under very difficult circumstances. Their comments are summarised in table 10.1.

The new approach to the preparation for the role of supervisor of midwives, and the widespread use of the open learning pack in particular, had a major impact on the quality of supervision in England. The new supervisors approached the role with an improved knowledge base, and the pack offered the means of achieving greater consistency in both the frameworks and practices in supervision.

The Board's *Midwifery Practice Audit* (ENB, 1997) revealed that supervision of midwives was gaining a higher profile in many maternity services. The increasing numbers of supervisors gave midwives better access and enriched the range of expertise available as the local teams of supervisors included clinical midwives, managers, educationalists and midwives in specialist roles.

Through the work of local teams of supervisors and the influence of the LSA responsible officers, many developments took place in supervision during the 1990s (Mayes, 1995). It was evident, however, that there were still issues which needed to be addressed such as the tension between the approach of newly appointed supervisors had the traditional approach of the existing supervisors. In some areas there were instances of poor supervision and inappropriate action taken by supervisors. In addition, changes to legislation and developments within the health service soon rendered the open learning pack out of date, as had been identified by the midwives who contributed to the Board's evaluation.

The development of the new programme

From 1993, when the first open learning programme was introduced, new demands and expectations were imposed on supervisors as the implementation of national initiatives influenced midwifery practice. Two important conferences took place in 1994 and 1995 which were to have a bearing on the evolution of supervision.

Table 10.1 Users' Views on the Experiences of Open Learning

The experience of open learning	
Positive aspects of the preparation	Aspects which could be improved
Flexibility to fit around other commitments	Inadequate study leave – very demanding on own time
Like to feel in control – used to organising own workloads	Clear information needed on what is required, especially for assessment
Confidence building	Need for regular feedback and reinforcement
Problem-solving approach felt to be appropriate for supervisors of midwives	Need for consistency in advice
Able to plan study to achieve most effective learning	Access to mentor/tutor counsellor
Own environment for study more conducive	Opportunity for peer discussion and networking
Retain all learning materials for future reference	Long distances to travel to study days, mentor and tutor
Able to use materials for teaching others	
Possible for several participants to be seconded from the workplace	

In October 1994, the UKCC held a working conference on the supervision of midwives involving participants from across the United Kingdom. The purpose was to identify and discuss the strengths and weaknesses of statutory supervision in order to inform the Midwifery Committee Task Group in developing standards for supervision. As a result, changes to the *Midwives Rules* were proposed which aimed to strengthen supervision and achieve consistency across the UK. The proposals were disseminated for consultation in 1995 and in 1997 Rule 44 was amended in legislation (SI no. 1723, 1997) to specify the educational requirements for supervisors of midwives. These included the learning outcomes for the programmes of preparation.

Table 10.2 Users' Views on the ENB Open Learning Pack

The Open Learning Pack	
Positive aspects of the preparation	Aspects which could be improved
Excellent!	Did not receive the pack on time
Enjoyable – even taken on holiday!	Difficulty in obtaining the 1979 Nurses, Midwives and Health Visitors Act
Kept to hand at all times for reference	
Comprehensive – everything needed for the course and for practice as a supervisor	Needs updating
Mix of activities and text – maintains interest	Would like more activities and examples – learnt most from them
Explanation following activities never leave issues unresolved	
Activities believable and relate to own practice areas – bringing the programme alive	
Grounded in practice throughout	
Approach inspiring – changed concept of supervision	

In 1995, another important conference took place, this one organised by the Association of Radical Midwives, entitled 'Super-Vision'. Presentations gave vivid accounts of midwives' experiences of the damaging effects of poor supervision. Other speakers offered insights into supervision in other professions (ARM, 1995). This stimulated debate and consideration of how to achieve more effective ways of enabling midwives to improve their practice and achieve professional development through the supervisory mechanism.

The nature of statutory supervision was developing rapidly at this time with supervisors emerging from the new programmes keen to introduce a new style of supervision. The importance of the approach of the supervisor in addition to the knowledge base on influencing the outcomes of supervising activities was gaining recognition. The proposals for clinical supervision (UKCC, 1995), although directed towards nursing and health visiting, offered some valuable insights for supervision of midwives. In particular, the potential of the partnership approach between supervisor and supervisee, providing a safe setting for reflecting on practice in order to achieve professional growth, was acknowledged.

Influenced by these considerations, a new culture was emerging in some units, which emphasised the supportive role of the supervisor of midwives. Alongside this was the desire for supervision to be proactive in facilitating good practice rather than reactive (concentrating on dealing with poor practice).

The requirement of the government for maternity services to provide woman centred care (NHSE, 1994) as promoted in the *Changing Childbirth* report recommendations, generated many implications for both midwives and their supervisors. These ranged from supporting midwives in their professional development to gain the competence and confidence to practise in new roles, to addressing the professional consequences of supporting women in exercising choice when those choices contravened trust policy or were inconsistent with the evidence for best practice.

As frameworks for risk management became established, clear parallels with supervision were apparent. Most supervising activities are consistent with the aims of risk management while retaining the unique characteristics of the professional function. In many maternity services, supervisors of midwives played an important part in implementing and participating in risk management strategies. In other cases, risk management was implemented in a controlling and restrictive fashion, rather than using evidence as the basis for guidelines to inform decision making.

In March 1996 the structures for supervision of midwives underwent change as a result of the relocation of the LSA function to the health authorities (Health Authority Act 1995; Nurses, Midwives and Health Visitors Act 1997). The most significant outcome of this move was the work achieved by the LSA responsible officers in collaboration with local maternity services. Each of the 12 consortia of LSAs appointed an experienced practising midwife as the responsible officer to undertake the work associated with the LSA function. The LSA responsible officers have since become a very influential group, providing midwifery leadership, monitoring the performance of local supervisory frameworks and contributing to strategic and contracting planning.

It was clear that these influences had to be reflected in the new open learning pack to enable supervisors of midwives to operate effectively and lead the development of practice within the context of the maternity services for the future. Consequently, the work involved far more than updating the sections on legislation as had been envisaged initially. It was agreed that the strengths of the first programme should be built upon, to ensure that the core purpose of providing a clear foundation for undertaking the role was maintained. The revision to the programme also offered the opportunity to develop the notion of the potential of supervision for supporting innovation in midwifery practice and empowering midwives who would give high quality, appropriate care within new models and innovative service frameworks.

To achieve such wide-ranging and visionary changes to the programme it was vital to draw upon the expertise of experienced supervisors of midwives, LSA responsible officers, midwives in clinical practice and midwifery educationalists to contribute to the work.

The new open learning programme

The work on updating the open learning programme involved a thorough revision. The content was reviewed for continued relevance, and those sections which had outlived their usefulness were removed. Most of the material which was to be retained was rewritten to update the language, and was rearranged into four new modules. New text was incorporated to ensure that the programme would equip supervisors for their responsibilities arising from the new national and service developments. Feedback from the users of the first pack had drawn attention to the value of the activities in achieving effective learning. In response to this, more activities and scenarios were compiled for inclusion in the text to reinforce essential points.

The programme was arranged in four modules representing the key components of the supervisor's role. Guidance on 'getting the most from this programme' was set out at the beginning of each module and made it clear that the modules need not be studied in any particular order.

MODULE 1:
Supervision and You: What is your role?

This module explores the role of the supervisor and, for those who begin with this module, it sets the scene for the more complex issues in supervision covered by the other modules. In establishing a clear understanding of the role, the main responsibilities are listed, and attention is drawn to the components of that role through acting as an expert practitioner, an educationalist, a manager, a leader and a researcher.

The issue of moving the focus of supervision away from a controlling negative influence, towards a proactive empowering role is introduced. It follows that, as the focus for midwifery care is that it is woman centred, the supervisor's perspective is midwife centred. Readers are encouraged to develop their personal vision of supervision.

MODULE 2:
Your Statutory Role and Organisational Models for Supervision

Module 2 examines the statutory basis for supervision, the primary legislation and the new *Rules*. This is the very foundation of supervision, and supervisors are required to have a thorough working knowledge of the rules and codes.

The supervisory framework is described and the interface with the LSA responsible officer is explored. Local systems for supervision are considered, such as the process for the nomination and appointment of supervisors. Every midwife must have access to a named supervisor at all times and the different ways of achieving this are discussed. The merits of midwives being able to choose their supervisor themselves are outlined, as compared with other systems such as allocation of midwives to a supervisor who is not their manager, systems which link the supervisor/manager role, or rotating the allocation to supervisors.

MODULE 3: Supporting Good Midwifery Practice

This is the longest of the modules, with the content divided into seven sections. It incorporates the topics presented in modules 2 and 4 of the first open learning programme, and because of the degree to which the supervisor's role in supporting good practice and professional development were inter-related, they have been combined in the same module.

The focus of the module is the approach of the supervisor in developing the quality of the relationship with midwives. The concept of supervision being increasingly seen as a supportive function is reinforced, and the benefits of achieving effective proactive relationships rather than reactive supervision are highlighted.

It is necessary for supervisors to have a clear understanding of accountability, and this section looks at how supervision can facilitate and empower midwives to exercise full accountability. Bergman's framework (Bergman, 1981) is used to demonstrate that midwives need confidence in their ability to practise safely so they can accept the responsibility and gain the necessary authority to act as accountable professionals. The importance of evidence to support good practice and professional responsibility is set out. This is developed to show how evidence-based practice provides a foundation for developing clinical guidelines and standards for practice, and how standards form the basis for auditing quality.

A new section on risk management has been included to demonstrate the key role which supervisors have to play. The process of risk management is examined and the links between supervision and risk management are identified. While supervision is a form of risk management in its own right and consequently supports local risk management systems, it is important to remember that the actions of the risk manager, the line manager and the supervisor of midwives are complementary but each has a separate and distinctive focus.

The section entitled 'Supervision in Practice' looks at how supervisors can assist midwives in relating their practice to the statutory requirements in the UKCC rules and codes. This includes reflecting on the complexities of interpreting the rules and professional standards in order to give appropriate advice and support.

The value of the annual supervisory review is discussed and examples of suitable documentation are presented. The reader is taken through the process of the review and consideration is given to how to get the most from the review. This leads on to how the supervisor can support midwives working outside the NHS.

The module ends by exploring the supervisor's role in professional development. Consideration is given to how the supervisor can empower midwives in their professional practice through facilitating professional development and using that development to inform organisational practices and policies. A range of activities takes readers through a process of using personal construct laddering to determine the characteristics of the supervisor they would like to be.

MODULE 4: Managing Professional Conduct

The last module is the most challenging, in that it is in this area that the fundamental tensions within the supervisory role lie. This programme has emphasised the supportive approach of enabling midwives to achieve high standards of practice as the means of protecting the public from unsafe practice. When mistakes occur or inappropriate decisions are made, the incident can be viewed as a learning opportunity. With support and respect from the supervisor, the midwife can reflect on the incident and hopefully will be receptive in learning from the experience in order to achieve a more appropriate standard of practice in the future. The dilemma is that the primary legislation places a duty on LSAs to investigate prima facie cases of alleged misconduct. In the interest of protecting the public, the investigation must be seen to be unbiased, fair and objective. This more distant, objective approach risks alienating the midwife, and jeopardising a potential learning opportunity. Dealing with cases of possible misconduct is a real test of the supervisor's skill and sensitivity.

The module discusses how the supervisor can identify a prima facie case, linking the misconduct to relevant rules and codes of practice or codes of professional conduct. Guidance is provided on points to consider when determining whether an investigation is needed and whether the case should be reported by the LSA to the UKCC. It leads on through the guiding principles of the planning and content of each stage of the investigation process.

In the interests of clarity the process of the investigation has been outlined to illustrate the principles which should be taken into account. As a result the process appears to mirror a disciplinary investigation. In reality, the supervisor's investigation may be less formal, and may take the form of the supervisor assisting the midwife to reflect on her practice, and agree the action plan together.

The use of the revised open learning programme

The new open learning programme has been in use since June 1997. Thirteen universities have been approved to deliver the programme of preparation for supervisors of midwives and the programme outcomes are assessed at the level of higher education diploma, degree or Masters level study. In addition to the midwives accessing the formal programme of preparation, many supervisors of midwives have purchased the pack for their own use as reference material, and many packs have been purchased for use by staff in maternity services.

When the pack had been in use for a year an evaluation was undertaken by the Board. The purpose of the evaluation was to identify:

- how effective the programme is for preparing midwives for undertaking the role of supervision of midwives
- how the programme is being used by different groups of midwives
- the future role of the Board in the preparation of supervisors of midwives.

There were two elements to the evaluation, which consisted of a questionnaire survey and four focus group discussions.

The questionnaires were sent to a sample of 229 midwives selected at random from student supervisors, mentor supervisors, programme leaders, approved midwife teachers, LSA responsible officers and heads of midwifery. There was a 51% response rate to the questionnaire, and 32 midwives attended the focus groups.

The findings demonstrate that the open learning programme has been well received by the target audience, the midwives undergoing preparation for the role, and it is also valued and used regularly by existing supervisors. There is evidence that the programme has led to a changed understanding of statutory supervision with support for a more proactive approach. The need for regular updating was highlighted to ensure that changes in legislationand so on are accommodated. The questionnaires sent to the student supervisors asked them to rate the usefulness of the programme in achieving the learning outcomes specified in Rule 44 of the *Midwives Rules*. These learning outcomes were introduced after the programme had been developed. Over 90% of respondents found the programme very useful or useful in relation to each of the Rule 44 outcomes.

The evaluation has shown that the Board's contribution to achieving effectiveness of supervision through the development of the open learning programme is valued. There was a consistent message throughout the work calling for the Board's involvement to continue in order to maintain the national perspective.

The future

The long-term future for supervision is uncertain. *The Review of the Nurses, Midwives and Health Visitors Act* by JM Consulting (JM Consulting, 1998) supports the continuation of supervision and the LSA function, influenced by the midwives' responses in the consultation process. This is endorsed in the Government (NHSE, 1999) response although it is suggested that the arrangements for statutory supervision may change as clinical governance develops.

An important feature of the Government's proposals for clinical governance (NHSE, 1999) is effective professional self-regulation. Statutory supervision of midwives has demonstrated its effectiveness in enabling midwives to maintain continuing fitness to practise beyond the point of registration. Evidence for this is the very small number of midwives who are called to appear before the Professional Conduct Committee at the UKCC. Supervision therefore has an important contribution to offer in clinical governance, and a similar mechanism would need to be introduced if statutory supervision were to be discontinued.

Until such time as the responsibility for professional regulation of nurses, midwives and health visitors is handed over to the new statutory body, the Nursing and Midwifery Council, the ENB will continue to produce the open learning programme for the preparation of supervisors of midwives. The Board will also support the LSA midwifery officers and supervisors of midwives in ensuring that there are robust frameworks for actively promoting safe standards of midwifery practice as our legacy to the new regulatory framework. This is particularly important as a means of securing a midwifery voice within trusts and providing effective midwifery leadership while midwifery management is becoming increasingly disempowered. Perhaps the leadership role of the supervisor is an aspect of the open learning programme which deserves further development if the pack is revised again.

The government's agenda for the 'New NHS' will bring many changes to midwifery practice and primary care groups offer exciting opportunities for innovative approaches to providing community-based maternity services, and health improvement programmes. The Commission for Health Improvement and the national service frameworks may well have implications for the context in which midwives practise. There will be important work for supervisors in enabling midwives to maintain their fitness to practise in new practice settings and in new roles. While some aspects of the open learning programme are already out of date, it will remain an invaluable resource for supervisors in undertaking this demanding role.

References

Bergman, R. (1981). 'Accountability – Definition and Dimensions'. *International Nursing Review* Vol. 28, No. 2, pp. 53-59.

Central Midwives Board (1939). *Rules*. Fourteenth Edition. London: CMB.

Department of Health (1993a). *Changing Childbirth: Report of the Expert Maternity Group*. London: HMSO.

ENB (1997). *Preparation of Supervision of Midwives*. London ENB.

ENB (1997). *Report of Midwifery Practice Audit 1996-1997*. London: ENB.

ENB (1992). *Preparation of Supervisors of Midwives – Supporting Good Midwifery Practice and Professional Development*. London: ENB.

Health Authorities Act 1995. London: HMSO.

JM Consulting Ltd (1998). *The Regulation of Nurses, Midwives and Health Visitors. Report on a Review of the Nurses, Midwives and Health Visitors Act 1997*. Bristol: JM Consulting.

Jenkins, R. (1995). *The Law and the Midwife*. Oxford: Blackwell.

Kirkham, M. (1995). 'The History of Midwifery Supervision'. In: ARM (Ed.) *Super-Vision Consensus Conference Proceedings*. Hale: Books for Midwives Press.

Mayes, G. (1995). 'Supervision of Midwives in 1995'. In: ARM (Ed.) *Super-Vision Consensus Conference Proceedings*. Hale: Books for Midwives Press.

Ministry of Health (1937). Circular 1620 *Supervision of Midwives*.

NHS Executive (1999). *Clinical Governance – Quality in the New NHS*. Leeds: NHSE.

NHS Management Executive (1994). EL(94)9 *Woman-centred Maternity Services*. Leeds: NHSME.

Nurses Midwives and Health Visitors Act 1997. London: The Stationery Office.

Statutory Instrument (1977) No. 1580. *The Midwives (Qualifications of Supervisors) Regulations*. London: HMSO.

Statutory Instrument (1997) No 1723. *The Nurses Midwives and Health Visitors (Supervisors of Midwives) Amendment Rules*. Approval Order 1997. London: HMSO.

UKCC (1995). Registrars Letter 4/1995 *Clinical Supervision for Nurses and Health Visitors*. London: UKCC.

UKCC (1998). *Midwives Rules*. London: UKCC.

Cathy Rogers • Chris Hallworth

Supervision at Masters Level
Development of a Preparatory Course

EDUCATION FOR SUPERVISORS

Learning to be a supervisor is not just about undertaking a course or doing the job, it is learning a new way of being yourself.
(Adapted from Claxton, 1978)

In May 1996 an item for discussion on the agenda of the Professional Midwifery Advisory Network (PMAN Group of the English National Board) centred on the 'Preparation of Supervisors of Midwives' open learning pack.

The question of assessment and accreditation led to a lively debate. As a member of the PMAN group I proposed setting this preparation course in a Masters pathway.

I emerged from that debate in a minority of one. As the chair concluded, I heard a quiet reflective voice of the then assistant director for supervision and practice say, 'The Board would always consider a proposal for such a course should one ever be presented'.

This postgraduate course in supervision of midwives was the first one to be presented to the Board, in December of that same year.

Rationale for development

Throughout the twentieth century the roles, functions and the education of the supervisor of midwives have been developed, redefined and honed as changes in the practice and the professional role of midwifery have altered. Supervisors are now required to provide both professional support and leadership for midwives (Steene 1995, ENB 1996, 1997). The ability of supervisors to provide professional leadership and support excellence in practice will to a large extent depend on their preparation for their role. As leadership deals with the future, supervisors need to be prepared with the necessary vision and appropriate skills to meet the needs of midwives and mothers in an ever-changing health care environment.

Since 1992 the preparatory course for supervisors of midwives has followed a more prescribed framework of study using the English National Board's open learning modules (ENB, 1997). Institutions that have delivered these programmes have required the midwife to undertake formal assessments and some have offered academic credits for appropriate achievement (Thomas and Mayes, 1996). These new educational programmes have had a positive impact both on the quality and profile of supervision. This was evident in Duerden's study in 1995 which concluded that supervision was 'alive and well' (Duerden, 1996). Her findings were in marked contrast to an earlier study in 1992 which reported that the profile of supervision in hospital was low and in the main centred on checking drugs and records (Allis, 1992). Moreover the new preparatory programme has been welcomed by supervisors, giving them more confidence in executing their role (Thomas and Mayes, 1996, Duerden, 1996). The scheme team shared the view that further improvements in practice would be evident with more advanced preparation for the role.

The need for this was supported by evidence from publications, audits and research which indicated that supervisors of midwives need to be more proactive in providing professional leadership for midwives and being catalysts for change in today's maternity care. The flattening of the maternity service structures, the ongoing changes in the organisation and provision of maternity care, and the challenges of providing women centred care have placed increasing demands on the role of the supervisor to provide an effective midwifery voice at all levels to ensure the ultimate goal of protection of the public. (Rogers 1993, Duerden 1995, 1996, Mayes 1995, 1996, Kirkham 1996). We saw it as vital that if supervisors are prepared to meet these challenges then they should be given appropriate academic recognition for their role and responsibilities. These views provided the foundation for the development of the postgraduate Certificate in the Supervision of Midwives which would give new supervisors an opportunity to prepare for that role at Masters level.

This development was also informed by the PREP framework for advanced practice (UKCC, 1994). The guidelines for advanced practice suggested that it was an important field of practice concerned with the continuing development of professionals and practice in the interests of patients and clients (UKCC, 1994). The advanced practitioner was to act as a consultant and policy maker and be a catalyst for change to improve professional standards and practice. Education for that role was to be at Masters level. The guidelines for advanced practice and the requirements of the advanced practitioner were congruent with the ENB's guidance to supervisors of midwives on their role and responsibilities (ENB 1996, 1997).

The supervisor of midwives, as an advanced practitioner, is required to utilise a wide variety of professional judgements and decision making skills that are contextualised within a range of practice environments. The ability to synthesise new knowledge, interpret evidence and advise others on the implications of health care strategies and policies are qualities expected to be demonstrated in practice (UKCC, 1994). This expert practitioner operates highly refined reflective practice skills in order to maintain and develop further excellence in practice.

Masters level study requires practitioners to undertake focused and in-depth analysis and critical evaluation creating, as a result, a more detailed insight into and understanding of the issues explored. Mastery implies the importance of contextualising data upon which professional judgements and decisions are made which are supported by enhanced communication skills in negotiation, collaboration, advocacy and empowerment, all of which are qualities essential for supervisory practice. It was felt that these are best addressed using academic skills commensurate with advanced level study.

Supported by two of our local supervising authority midwifery responsible officers a decision was made to prepare some of their nominated supervisors of midwives at Masters level leading to the award of Postgraduate Certificate in the Supervision of Midwives (Pg Cert).

Conscious of the fact that the main function of the role of supervisor remains the protection of the public, the views and expectations of the users of our maternity services were sought. Using the Association for Improvements in the Maternity Services, who are familiar with the midwifery statutory framework, and through the chair of this group, the scheme team were well informed about the difficulties and expectations of families as they negotiate the maternity services.

Postgraduate Certificate in Supervision

With a commitment to preparing supervisors of midwives at Masters level who would emerge as professional leaders, the course team prepared a framework to develop the personal, intellectual, reflective and practice skills of those nominated. In order to achieve a Postgraduate Certificate in the Supervision of Midwives students would have to complete the following three courses:

- Course One: The Practice of Midwifery Supervision
- Course Two: Skills to Support Midwifery Supervision
- Course Three: Supervision of Midwives in Action – The Management of Midwifery Supervision

On successful completion of Courses One and Two midwives who have been nominated by the local supervising authority are recommended as eligible for appointment as a supervisor by the local supervising authority. To achieve the academic award of Postgraduate Certificate in the Supervision of Midwives, supervisors must complete Course Three. This course can be studied only after a minimum of 20 weeks in practice as a supervisor, thus enabling supervisors to bring to their studies contemporary issues which they wish to analyse, evaluate and synthesise. The course is also open to experienced supervisors as a statutory refresher course.

Course One: The Practice of Midwifery Supervision

This course attracts 30 academic credits and is delivered over a 20-week period. The role, functions, values and place of midwifery supervision are the key focus of this course, in addition to exploring a selection of models and frameworks for executing the role in practice. The course explores contemporary issues impacting on maternity care and the role of the supervisor in providing professional leadership for midwives and supporting excellence in practice. The complementary but conflicting aspects of clinical supervision and midwifery supervision are addressed in order to establish the differences and value of each. Models and frameworks for professional judgements and decision making are explored, how these may be used by supervisors to implement the statutory framework governing the supervision of midwives. In addition, the role of the supervisor in supporting evidence-based practice, facilitating clinical audit and risk management are developed.

Course Two: Skills to Support Midwifery Supervision

This course attracts 15 academic credits and is delivered over a 20-week period in conjunction with Course One. The key focus in this course is on the development of the skills necessary to advance practice including assertiveness, negotiation and conflict management skills. Skills such as advocacy, empowerment and communication are also addressed. Workshops are provided to facilitate reflection and critical evaluation by the nominee of their personal performance in use of these skills.

The modules which make up the open learning study packs provided by the ENB are incorporated throughout these courses. (ENB, 1997). Students are provided with guidance on using the open learning material but are responsible for planning their study time to complete these.

Course Three: Supervision of Midwives in Action – The Management of Midwifery Supervision

This course attracts 15 academic credits and is delivered over a 12-week period. This course explores the theoretical and practice issues of concern to supervisors who aim to advance practice in the context of contemporary influences impacting on their role. Learning contracts are used, enabling supervisors to direct their studies on a contemporary issue they wish to analyse, evaluate and synthesise.

Practice development requirements for Courses One and Two

For the duration of these courses students are linked to an experienced supervisor who acts as their mentor. The students regularly meet with their mentor for a nominal hour of contact each week structured for feedback and appraisal about their development. In addition students are required to schedule a minimum of four hours per week to focus in practice on the role and responsibilities of supervisors of midwives. During this period of focused practice students are required to negotiate with their mentor participation, reflection and critical evaluation on the role of the supervisors in relation to staff development and support, clinical audit, risk management, standard setting and policy review and development.

Students are required to submit in their portfolio of practice experiences a critical analysis and evaluation of how supervision functions in their unit in relation to these activities, alongside their recommendations for future developments. This provides students with an opportunity to demonstrate the integration of theory with practice and to analyse the strengths and weaknesses of the model of supervision in their own practice site.

Generally the evaluations indicate that the role of the supervisor in relation to the above key responsibilities needs to be more clearly defined and strengthened if supervisors are to provide professional leadership and support excellence in practice. It is also worth noting the wide variation and interpretation that exists in different units as to the role of the supervisor in these areas. This needs proper evaluation and the development of clearer standards and frameworks for supervisors.

During this period of focused practice students also have the opportunity to visit other units and undertake a comparative analysis of different models of supervision. In addition they are encouraged to visit private sector hospitals, general practitioners' practices and independent midwives to evaluate how supervision functions in different settings. These experiences are negotiated through their practice mentor and positively contribute to the students' development, giving them a broader insight into their role.

A further requirement of students during their practice placement is to observe and participate in a minimum of five interviews with midwives in their own unit. This gives students an opportunity to analyse the interpersonal skills used to facilitate the interview and empower midwives as autonomous practitioners.

The portfolio is a course requirement and contributes to both the formative and summative elements of the course. The commitment and motivation of the mentors in providing support and guidance for the students is central to their development. The selection and preparation of mentors to undertake this role is paramount. Practice mentors are briefed on the philosophy of the courses, the programme of studies, assessment strategies and the enormous commitment requested of them. All practice mentors are issued with a handbook and are linked to a university lecturer for support and guidance. Recognition of their contribution is provided for their own professional portfolio.

Teaching and learning strategies

In order to achieve the aims and outcomes of the programme the teaching and learning strategies are designed to facilitate active participation and are based on the principles of adult learning (Kolb 1984, Burnard 1985, Ramsden 1992, Reid and Proctor 1993). In view of the supervisor's responsibilities for promoting autonomous practice it is important that teaching and learning activities are modelled on this philosophy.

A variety of teaching strategies are used which support the development of the practice and intellectual skills required to function in the role. These include problem based learning approaches, experiential workshops, simulation and role plays based on practice dilemmas, peer teaching, case reviews and seminar presentations.

Using these experiences provides a good opportunity for the nominated supervisor to experience demanding situations in a safe environment with the benefits of developing skills that are transferable in practice. These approaches are supported with appropriate guidance and support from the academic staff.

In addition to these strategies a number of key lectures are incorporated into the programme, which support the student centred learning activities. These include lectures on:

- judgement and decision making
- decision trees and utilities
- models and frameworks for supervision
- concepts of autonomy and advocacy
- risk management
- leadership and change theory
- theory of motivation and empowerment.

Key sessions are also provided by senior midwifery managers who address the political factors impacting on midwifery and supervision alongside the challenges facing supervisors of the future.

The students are given the opportunity to meet with professional officers from the statutory bodies including the responsible midwifery officers which provides a discussion forum for the presentation of specialist knowledge led by experts in the field.

The content of these study days builds upon the ENB distance learning material which forms the self-directed teaching component of the courses. The students are required to submit evidence of having studied their distance learning texts in their portfolio of practice development.

As students of the postgraduate school here at the University of Hertfordshire, nominated supervisors have access to the integrated learning resources centre which provides access to computing, library and media services. The centre is open 24 hours Monday to Friday during term-time and from 1100 hrs to 2300 hrs at weekends. Sessions on evidence-based practice to support the development of judgement and decision making skills in practice are undertaken in the computing laboratories where students have hands-on experience supported by midwifery lecturers and consultants of the learning resources centre. The multi-media studios provide an ideal venue to facilitate workshop and simulation activities for developing the skills to support them in their practice. These provisions have been positively evaluated by the students.

Assessment strategy

As the learning outcomes of the programme require evidence of high intellectual ability and mastery in skills of communication, negotiation, advocacy and empowerment then it follows that the assessment strategy should enable such skills to be demonstrated.

The assessment methods comprised an incremental case study, a portfolio of practice and a video interview with 20 minutes of discussion with practice assessors, one being an LSA midwifery officer and the other an academic supervisor of midwives who elicit the achievements made by the nominated supervisor.

Presentation of the assessment strategy created an academic debate on how assessors could determine higher level ordered skills in practice other than by the written word that would stand up to scrutiny.

The scheme team were determined that the assessment would echo the philosophy and primacy of practice of midwifery supervision and not the theoretical exposition of the statutory role.

In determining the assessment strategy the supervisors of midwives on the scheme team and the LSA midwifery officers were adamant that the methods of assessment focus upon practice skills which supervisors of midwives use regularly, providing a valuable framework of experience for future use within the role.

In addition the strategy reflects the qualities of advanced level academic and practice performance which are considered essential for the supervisors of midwives in contemporary midwifery practice. As a key leader of the midwifery profession, the supervisor of midwives needs to have the ability and expertise to articulate and discuss complex and contextualised practice issues in a variety of forums.

Evidence shows that the learning outcomes for Course One were achieved by using an incremental case study approach. Students are presented with allegations and reports on an investigation. They are required to analyse and discriminate the evidence in respect of contemporary practice and to contextualise the evidence, demonstrating a reasoned, critical argument in respect of the professional judgements made in the report. A synthesis of the evidence recommendations is made, from which a policy and rationale is developed.

Assessment of the learning outcomes for Course Two requires the student to undertake a video recorded role play interview which specifically focuses upon the proactive role of the supervisor of midwives in enhancing and improving the quality of care. The aim is to provide, through role play interview and discussion, evidence of their ability to undertake supervisory activity using the intellectual abilities itemised above and take a leadership role within the profession. This assessment is designed to measure the students' ability to use skills in negotiation, advocacy, leadership and empowerment to facilitate changes in practice or collaboration within a multiprofessional environment.

In addition, the student's ability to motivate, inspire and challenge the ideas and assumptions of others, including proposing alternative management options, are key qualities assessed. They are required to demonstrate a non-judgmental attitude and display empathy and political awareness. Immediately following the role play, the student undertakes a discussion with the two assessors which provides the opportunity to clarify the rationale for their decisions, judgements and actions and their structure and approach to the interview.

The role plays may be between a supervisor of midwives (the student) and a midwife, a mother, a purchaser or a provider of health care and reflect the wide variety of situations that the supervisor will have to interface with in practice. These roles are undertaken by midwifery lecturers, with two practice assessors observing and assessing the role play.

Students are provided with their scenario 15 minutes prior to undertaking the role play. Any notes the student wishes to make during this time may be taken to the role play. The role play lasts between 25 to 35 minutes at the most. All students are debriefed following the role play and discussion by an experienced midwifery lecturer.

From appointment to completion

On successful completion of Courses One and Two, comprising the preparation course, the nominated supervisor of midwives is eligible to be appointed. The LSA midwifery officers who are members of the board of examiners receive the results and a report on the development of their nominee. They also scrutinise the portfolios of practice development to ensure the nominee has had the requisite experiences in practice. In some instances a further period of experience is considered appropriate before appointment but the majority are appointed within a month following publication of the examination board results.

Following a minimum of six months in the role as supervisors of midwives the final course comprising the award of the Postgraduate Certificate in the Supervision of Midwives (Pg Cert), 'Supervision of Midwives in Action – The Management of Midwifery Supervision' is completed supported by five contact study days over a twelve week period. The assessment method for Course Three is by coursework with the presentation of a portfolio. The aim is to provide a framework for supervisors to undertake an in-depth enquiry into contemporary issues impacting on their role.

The assessment requires the midwife to negotiate a learning contract which identifies the practice issue they wish to study. Evidence of achievement is presented by portfolio. This may be in the form of annotated bibliographies with discussion on the validity and reliability of the evidence presented, records and reflective accounts of attendance at an alternative area to observe different practices, or an essay which critically evaluates the evidence found and determines how practices should evolve. In their portfolio students are required to demonstrate the intellectual ability to discriminate, synthesise and contextualise the evidence appropriate for contemporary practice, demonstrating incisive and reasoned critical argument and advanced professional judgements.

The component parts of the assessment strategy therefore require the midwife to explore very specific aspects of the role of supervisors of midwives. The opportunity is given for the midwife to undertake an in-depth critical evaluation of the research and other supportive evidence for midwifery practice together with the requirement to seek new solutions and proposals for future practice.

Fears were expressed by some members of the profession that setting a course at Masters level would deter many motivated midwives from applying, fearing they would be unable to study at this level. This, however, has not been borne out: the numbers nominated for each cohort has increased. The current cohort has 20 undertaking the preparation course, all at postgraduate level.

The external examiner's reports have highlighted the sound knowledge, insight and advanced interpersonal skills achieved by the student supervisors, demonstrated through the innovatory and entirely appropriate assessment methods. The students and the team were complimented on the high standard achieved.

Evaluation

As this initiative is new, ongoing evaluation is a crucial element in the delivery of the course. The current evaluation systems provide information on the student's experiences of the course, the programme of studies and the assessment strategies. Feedback is also available from the internal and external assessors and the student nominated LSA officers. As with any new programme the most important element to inform future developments is its impact on the practice of supervision. This is the focus of a current audit which can be used to inform future educational programmes for the preparation of supervisors of midwives.

The development has been viewed positively by the midwives undertaking the initial preparation programmes (Courses One and Two) and the supervisors who have completed Course Three either for refresher purposes or to receive the award of the postgraduate certificate. Nevertheless, students expressed anxiety about the level of study and the assessment strategies and require ongoing encouragement, support and feedback from their personal tutors who are also supervisors of midwives.

Despite these anxieties, which are common to most courses and were evident when the ENB revised their preparation programmes in the 1990s (Thomas and Mayes, 1996), the majority of students have successfully achieved the outcomes of the courses at Level Four (Masters level).

To date, 48 nominated supervisors have enrolled for the preparation courses, 'The Practice of Midwifery Supervision and Skills to Support

Midwifery Supervision'. Of these, 26 have successfully completed, of whom 21 were successful at the first attempt with the remaining five being successful at the second. Two nominees have left the programme: one because of ill-health and one as a result of a change in career pathway. Twenty nominees are in the process of completing their preparation programme.

The academic profile of the nominees met the eligibility requirements for them to register for Masters level credits. Initially some students expressed anxiety at achieving the Masters level outcomes of these programmes and required reassurance and support from their personal tutor before making their final commitment. By the end of the preparation period the nominated supervisors were in agreement that the role and responsibilities that they had been prepared for were commensurate with advanced practice.

Student feedback questionnaire

The student feedback questionnaire is a three-part questionnaire. The first section addresses university-wide concerns. The second section, part B, concentrates on the courses studied. Students are asked to provide an overall rating for 33 statements focusing upon course content, course organisation and delivery, methods of teaching and learning and learning resources in addition to the course assessment strategies. The statements are rated from A to E, depending on students' level of agreement. An A rating implies 100 per cent agreement, B rating 80 per cent agreement, C rating 60 per cent agreement, D rating 40 per cent agreement and an E rating implies a 20 per cent agreement with the statement.

To date we have received 20 completed questionnaires from the students who have completed Courses One and Two, 'The Practice of Midwifery Supervision' and 'Skills to Support Midwifery Supervision'. The overall feedback from the students has been excellent, with 48 per cent of students awarding an A and 52 per cent a B for both courses. In response to the statement as to how well the courses prepared them to undertake the role of supervisor of midwives, 38 per cent awarded A, 59 per cent B and 3 per cent C.

Students are also asked for an evaluation of the appropriateness of the assessment strategy and its application to the practice of supervision.

FIGURE 11.1

TOTAL RESPONDENTS 51

Please indicate how useful you found the 4 modules to be:

	Very useful	Useful	Quite useful	Not useful
(i) Understand the ways in which the supervision of midwives enhances standards of care	53%	38%	4%	–
	91%			
(ii) Understand the application of law relevant to midwifery practice and the supervision of midwives	58%	38%	–	–
	96%			
(iii) Be able to provide professional support to practising midwives relevant to maintaining and promoting standards of care	51%	42%	4%	–
	93%			
(iv) Be able to encourage midwives to use their experience in practice to enhance their professional development	33%	56%	11%	–
	89%			
(v) Gain an understanding of accountability and professional responsibility as a supervisor of midwives (Registrars Letter 21/1997 UKCC)	58%	33%	9%	–
	91%			
(vi) Gain an awareness of the demands and challenges involved in supervision	60%	31%	4%	–
	91%			
(vii) Create a personal vision of the role of the supervisor of midwives	47%	36%	16%	–
	83%			
(viii) Relate supervision to current changes in the NHS that influence midwifery practice and supervision of midwives	29%	60%	6%	–
	89%			

Sixty per cent rated this statement as an A, 25 per cent B, 12 per cent C and 3 per cent D.

In addition to completing the questionnaire, students are asked to comment on the aspects of the courses they enjoyed most and least in addition to recommendations for further development. The most enjoyable aspects of the course which are most frequently commented on are the university contact study days, particularly the theoretical content of these days, participation in classroom activities, role plays and interaction with lecturers, supervisors and peer groups.

This has important implications for future preparation programmes as clearly there needs to be a satisfactory balance between the distance learning components and contact study days at the study centres. Indeed, the most frequent comments received under suggestions for future development are, more contact study days and, more contact with their personal tutor. In the context of these courses students value the opportunity, through role play and simulation, to explore their skills of advocacy, empowerment, negotiation, conflict management and leadership in a safe environment. The aspect of the course most frequently cited by students as least enjoyable was the travelling to the university!

Feedback from responsible officers

The evaluation and feedback from the local supervising authorities midwifery officers has greatly informed the quality and ongoing development of the programme. In their evaluations they 'wholeheartedly support the academic stringency of preparing would be supervisors at Masters level' (Truttero, 1999) and assert that this is the 'appropriate level of preparation given the demands of the role' (Kirby, 1999).

Whilst acknowledging our completely different approach to the preparation and assessment of new supervisors, they are firm in their belief that this should be the required level of preparation if the 'improvements we hope for supervision and practice are to be realised' (Kirby, 1999). The arguments they put to support their views include the move 'towards an all graduate profession', 'the impact of clinical governance' and the 'development of primary care groups' alongside the responsibility of the supervisor to provide 'effective midwifery leadership' (Kirby 1999, Truttero 1999). Indeed Truttero concludes that the future 'strategy for educationalists and LSA officers should be to increase the number of supervisors of midwives who can function at Masters level to secure the future of the profession'. To do otherwise she believes 'would be sacrificial' (Truttero, 1999).

In their evaluations they commend the achievement of the programme for the development and integration of the theory and principles of supervision with the practice of supervision and the emphasis given to the development and assessment of the practical skills required to function in the role (Kirby 1999, Truttero 1999).

Conclusion

Statutory supervision of midwives evolved in an environment of social conflict and confusion as to the role that midwives should play in maternity care (Donnisson 1988, Heagerty 1990, Rogers 1993). The model which predominated was viewed as punitive and constraining rather than facilitative or supportive (Heagerty 1990, Rogers 1993). Despite its historical origins, supervision has been retained as the process provides a statutory framework for professional support, leadership and the facilitation of autonomous practice (Rogers 1993, Mayes 1996, Thomas and Mayes 1996, ENB 1996, 1997). The importance of supervision in enabling midwifery practice is paramount. Supervisors of midwives should not only be able to demonstrate 'qualities of sympathy and tact', but be proactive in supporting excellence in practice and providing professional leadership (Rogers 1993, Mayes 1996).

Preparation for that role is vital, given the challenges facing midwives and the marginalisation of midwives at operational level. The first education programme for supervisors was introduced in 1978 comprising a two-day induction course to be completed in the first year of appointment. The programme for preparation was further developed by the ENB in 1992 and 1996 because of concern about the profile and quality of supervision in practice.

The Postgraduate Certificate in the Supervision of Midwives marks the further development in the preparation of supervisors, allowing would-be supervisors academic recognition and advanced preparation for their role and responsibilities. The overall feedback from the students and responsible officers suggests that this should be the level of preparation for future programmes, although the benefits of this level of preparation have to be determined in practice. We await with interest the outcome of the audit currently being performed by Eastern Region West, evaluating different approaches to the education of supervisors in order to inform future educational strategies. If this is the way forward then clearly there are implications for reviewing UKCC *Rule 44* which stipulates the minimum outcomes of preparatory programmes and are, in our view, incongruent with the requirements of the role.

Undoubtedly, the nature of supervision will continue to evolve as supervisors respond to contemporary influences impacting on maternity care and the commissioning and provision of maternity services. Moreover, the outcome of the recent review of the Nurses, Midwives and Health Visitors Act will have a major impact on the future of supervision and education for supervisors. If statutory supervision is to be retained, the key focus of all preparatory programmes is to support the development of the intellectual and practice skills required by supervisors to develop the frontiers of practice in the interests of mothers and babies.

Acknowledgements

In recognition of their contribution to the preparation and ongoing development of this course we would like to thank Kathie Bell, Joy Kirby and Suzanne Truttero our LSA midwifery officers, and Chris Lawrence, the Director of Studies at the University of Hertfordshire, for her support and speed in presenting this programme for validation.

References

Allis, P. (1992). Managing the Issues Relating to the Review, Development and Implementation of Supervision of Midwives. Unpublished dissertation (copy in RCM Library, London).

Burnard, P. (1985). *Learning Human Skills*. Oxford: Heinemann Medical Books.

Butterworth, T., Faugier, J. (eds.) (1992). *Clinical Supervision and Mentorship in Nursing*. London: Chapman and Hall.

Claxton, G. (1978). *The Little Ed Book*. London: Routledge and Regan.

Donnison, J. (1988). *Royal College of Midwives 'Midwives and Medical Men'*. London: Historical Publications.

Duerden, J. (1995). *Audit of Supervision of Midwives in the North West Regional Health Authority*. Salford: Salford Royal Hospitals NHS Trust.

Duerden, J. (1996). 'Auditing supervision: an example of one audit and general issues concerning audit'. In: Kirkham, M. (ed.) *Supervision of Midwives*. Hale: Books for Midwives Press.

ENB (1996). *Preparation of Supervisors of Midwives 'The English National Board's Advice and Guidance to Local Supervising Authorities and Supervisors of Midwives'*. London: ENB.

ENB (1995). *Preparation of Supervisors of Midwives 'Developments in Midwifery Education and Practice – A Progress Report'*. London: ENB.

ENB (1996). *Preparation of Supervisors of Midwives Midwifery Supervision: A New Perspective Conference Report*. London: ENB.

ENB (1997). *Preparation of Supervisors of Midwives (Module 1-4)* London: ENB.

Heagerty, B. (1990). Class, Gender and Professionalisation: the Struggle for British Midwifery 1900-1936. Unpublished PhD thesis, University of Michigan (copy in RCM Library, London).

Kirby, J. (1999). *Evaluation of Preparatory Course for Supervisors of Midwives*. Academic Quality Assurance, Hatfield: University of Hertfordshire.

Kirkham, M. (Ed) (1996). *Supervision of Midwives*. Hale: Books for Midwives Press.

Kolb, D. (1984). *Experiential Learning*. New Jersey: Prentice-Hall.

Mayes, G. (1995). 'Supervision of Midwives: How Can We Facilitate Change'. In *ENB Education Resource Pack*. London: ENB.

Mayes, G. (1996). 'The Changing Face of Supervision of Midwives'. *British Journal of Midwifery*, Vol. 4, No. 1, January.

Ramsden, P. (1992). *Learning in Higher Education*. London and New York: Routledge.

Reid, J. Proctor, S. (1993). *Nurse Education: A Reflective Approach*. London: Arnold.

Rogers, C.A. (1993). Supervision of Midwives – A Practice Questioned. Unpublished MA dissertation, Middlesex University (copy in Middlesex University Library, Enfield).

Steene, J. (1995). 'Supervision of Midwives: Proposed Changes to the Midwives' Rules'. *British Journal of Midwifery*, Vol. 3, No. 9, September.

Steene, J. (1995). 'A Prominent Role for the Local Supervising Authority'. *British Journal of Midwifery*, Vol. 3, No. 6, June.

Thomas, M., Mayes, G. (1996). 'The ENB Perspective: Preparation of Supervisors of Midwives for their Role'. In: Kirkham, M. (ed) *Supervision of Midwives*. Hale: Books for Midwives Press.

Truttero, S. (1999). *Evaluation of Preparatory Course for Supervisors of Midwives*. Academic Quality Assurance, Hatfield: University of Hertfordshire.

UKCC (1994). *Standards for Education and Practice Following Registration*. London: UKCC.

INDEX